Adapting Chair Yoga
for Every Body

ADAPTING
CHAIR YOGA
for EVERY BODY

FINLAY WILSON

Forewords by Dr Emilia Ferraro and Cor Hutton
Photography by Alastair Wilson

SINGING DRAGON
LONDON AND PHILADELPHIA

First published in Great Britain in 2026 by Jessica Kingsley Publishers
An imprint of John Murray Press

1

The information contained in this book is not intended to replace the services of trained medical
professionals or to be a substitute for medical advice. The complementary therapy described in
this book may not be suitable for everyone to follow. You are advised to consult a doctor before
embarking on any complementary therapy programme and on any matters relating to your
health, and in particular on any matters that may require diagnosis or medical attention.

A CIP catalogue record for this title is available from the British Library and the Library of Congress

ISBN 978 1 80501 413 3
eISBN 978 1 80501 414 0

Printed and bound in Great Britain by CPI Group.

Jessica Kingsley Publishers' policy is to use papers that are natural, renewable and recyclable
products and made from wood grown in sustainable forests. The logging and manufacturing
processes are expected to conform to the environmental regulations of the country of origin.

Jessica Kingsley Publishers
Carmelite House
50 Victoria Embankment
London EC4Y 0DZ

www.jkp.com

John Murray Press
Part of Hodder & Stoughton Ltd
An Hachette Company

The authorised representative in the EEA is Hachette Ireland,
8 Castlecourt Centre, Dublin 15, D15 XTP3, Ireland (email: info@hbgi.ie)

Contents

Acknowledgments 9

Forewords by Dr Emilia Ferraro and Cor Hutton 11

PART ONE **Why Chair Yoga? Understanding the Fundamentals of an Accessible Yoga Practice**

CHAPTER 1 Introduction 17
A Note on Language and Cueing   23

CHAPTER 2 The Fundamentals 25
Structuring Your Practice   25
Props and Equipment   27
Basic Moves   28

PART TWO **Practices**

CHAPTER 3 Warming Up 33
Wrist Stretches – Finger Pulls   35
Wrist Extensor Stretch – Pour   35
Wrist Extensor Stretch – Curl   36
Cat   36
Cat Variations   37
Bow Pulls   38
Shoulder Flossing   38
Rear Deltoid Press   40
Neck Isometrics   40
Neck Rotations   42
Shoulder Shrugs   42
Active Archer   43
Eagle Arms Preparation   43
Eagle Arms Rotations   44
Eagle Arms   45

Kite Hawk   45
Dynamic Thoracic Twists   47
Bridge with a Roll   47
Side Bend with Neck Release   48
Neck Release (Following on from Side Bend)   48
Dynamic Hip Mobility Twist   49
Dynamic Block Step Overs   49
Dynamic Quad Extensions   51
Ankle Rotations and Point and Flex   52
Double Quad Extensions   52
Adductor Activation Presses   53
Abductor Activation Presses   53
Shoulder Reliever   54
Unlocking The Shoulders – Single Arm   54
Unlocking The Shoulders – Both Arms   55
Bird Wing   55
Weighted Shrugs   56

CHAPTER 4 Core Work 57
Abs with a Roll   58
Alternating Leg Lifts   58
Alternating Leg Lifts with Arm and Leg Extension   59
Oblique Crunch   59
Oblique Crunch in Horse   60
Navasana Prep   60
Navasana   61

CHAPTER 5 Forward Bends. 63
Forward Bend with a Blanket   64
Forward Bend with Blocks   65
Forward Bend with a Bolster   66
Halfway Lift on Blocks   66
Forward Bend with Neck Traction   67
Single Leg Hold with a Strap (Stage 1)   67
Thigh Adduction (Stage 2)   68
Thigh Abduction (Stage 3)   68
Twisting Triangle (Stage 4)   69
Standing Forward Bend   69
Active Standing Forward Bend   70
Single Leg Forward Bend   71
Pyramid   71

CHAPTER 6 Back Bends. 73
Chest Opening Pose   74
Single Arm Chest Opening   75
Neck Release   76
Neck Release (Arm Hold)   76
Dolphin   77

Bridge with a Roll 78
Chair Pose 78
Lunge 79
Chest Opener 80
Cactus Arms Back Bend 80
Chest Opener 81
Back Bend with a Strap 82
Strap Camel 82
Neck Traction 83
Reverse Tabletop 84
Dancer 84
Upward Facing Dog 85

CHAPTER 7   Twists 87
Active Twist 88
Twist 89
Twist with Hips 90
Active Twist with Wide Arms 90
Chair Pose Twist 1 91
Chair Pose Twist 2 92
Chair Pose Twist 3 92
Chair Pose Twist at the Wall 93
Dynamic Twist 94
Dynamic Twist with Neck Isometrics 94
Twisting Squat 1 95
Twisting Squat 2 96
Twisting Lunge 96
Twisting Triangle 97

CHAPTER 8   Standing Poses 99
Side Bend in Horse 100
Warrior 2 101
Reverse Warrior 102
Extended Warrior 102
High Lunge/Warrior 1 103
Twisting Warrior 104
Triangle 104
Knee to Chest 105
Back Release 106
Lunge Heel to Butt 106
Lunge Side Bend 107
Chair-Assisted Ankle Strengthener 1 108
Chair-Assisted Ankle Strengthener 2 108
Single Leg Balance 109
Warrior 3 109
Half Moon 110
Tree 111

CHAPTER 9   Dynamic Movement   113

     Sun Salutation A   114

     Classical Sun Salutation   116

     Sun Salutation A (Variation)   118

     Sun Salutation B   120

     Hip Circumduction   122

CHAPTER 10   Relaxing   125

     Restorative Single Leg Forward Bend   126

     Savasana   127

     Chest Opener Savasana   127

     Legs Up Savasana   127

     Supported Forward Bend   128

     Deluxe Savasana   128

CHAPTER 11   Breathwork   129

     Ujjayi Breathing   130

     Sitali   131

     Sitkari   132

     Bhramari   132

     Kapalabhati   132

     Full Yogic Breath   133

     Viloma   133

     Alternate Nostril Breathing   134

     Surya Bhedana   135

     Chandra Bhedana   135

     Anuloma   135

CHAPTER 12   Meditation   137

     Squeeze and Release   138

     Body Scanning   139

     Breath Counting   141

     Duality   142

PART THREE   Teaching Chair Yoga for Every Body

CHAPTER 13   Setting Up a Chair Yoga Class   147

CHAPTER 14   Sample Classes   151

     Short Practice: Upper Body   151

     Short Practice: Lower Body   152

     Short Practice: Everyday Sequence   152

     Long Practice: Twists   153

     Long Practice: Forward Bends   153

     Long Practice: Back Bends   154

     Long Practice: Dynamic Movement   155

Epilogue   157

Resources   160

Acknowledgments

Having been fortunate enough to travel all over the world to study history and study how people find connection with their environment, I have practised yoga in many different places and with many different people. I owe a debt of gratitude to the teachings from India and South Asia and the ways they have shaped my mind, my body and the healing arts that have been offered to me as I have developed as a teacher and bodyworker. I've stepped into lineages tracing back names that are tethered to a history and sharing that has gone on for a long time.

Through self-study and investigation, translation and fascination, I've delved into the texts of the ancients and indigenous peoples to absorb concepts of how to view the world, how to heal the body and the mysteries of the mind. I encourage you to explore these texts yourself and sit with them a while (*The Yoga Sutras of Patanjali*, *Hatha Yoga Pradipika*, *The Upanishads*, *The Ramayana* and *Light On Yoga* to name a few).

Looking back to when I first started teaching, I must thank my early students for their patience with my mistakes, fumbles and good intentions as I learned the difference between my own practice, their practice and the process of deconstructing the imposed rules of various systems I had been part of. I blush as I reflect, but that is all part of growth. I thank the trust shown by these early students of mine whose enthusiasm led me to pursue more information to better show up for them – a theme within the groups of people with whom I have worked throughout the years.

Thank you to my long-suffering twin brother, Alastair, for his dedication to photography and skill behind the lens. While it may not have been the path he thought he would go on, he has now become quite the prolific yoga photographer, assisting me on our second publication together. Three hundred poses in and numerous angle changes later, you need someone who can say without harm that you look a bit greasy and that maybe you should eat something. The laughs, as they always have done, come easily. If you want someone who is good with still or moving images, but who also knows when not to take the shot (an undervalued skill in photography), he is your guy!

I have so much gratitude for my family, and there are a lot of us. We saw throughout our childhood the care and compassion shown to our Great Uncle Bill Dryden (my maternal grandmother's brother) and Great Aunt Meg Morrison (my paternal grandmother's cousin), both amputees, and the exuberance that they both showed as a pervasive force in our formative years. I would also be remiss not to mention the stellar patience of my mother (Margaret Wilson) who has, even when I was younger, spoken to me of the many ways workplaces and institutions should be equal, accessible and diverse. My mum still stands as a reminder in her charity work with Healthy Valleys about the importance of connection, health and access, regardless of geographic or economic conditions.

To my husband, Alan. We met in the yoga room and most of our life is now spent in one. Together we guide and encourage, bringing a balance through the styles we teach, and as everyone always says, it's the dream team. Your management of the tangible studio side of the charity allows me to dream and plan a future that can lift people up and to design new programmes. Importantly, I thank you for chasing me back to the computer when I get distracted.

The idea for this book has been long in the making, but it was the beginning of a partnership with an amputee charity in Scotland that really kicked me into gear to get started. To the 'troops' at Finding Your Feet, we are now a few years into working together, our numbers are increasing and your resilience, determination and willingness to explore and be open with me have helped shape this book into a manual that I hope you will use, because it is all the good stuff that you know (and a fair smattering of the stuff you don't like, too).

To the charity, Heart Space. We have been at this for more than a decade together to the point that so many faces have changed and moved on that I guess I am dedicating this to the bricks and mortar. I remember walking through the wreck of a building, with plants growing on the inside, with both of my parents wide-eyed, and thinking I could never get the place ready, let alone open a yoga studio. But now, all these years later, we see hundreds of people every week entering that space, taking in the light through the stained-glass windows and finding a second home. With many late nights and early mornings, laughter and tears, you have become the foundation for all that I do. A dream, realised.

Forewords

I had practised yoga for many years before I had my prosthetic, and as soon as I got out of the hospital, I realised that I needed to do something to recognise this body that was a different body. I immediately thought, 'I need to do yoga.' The day after I had my prosthetic on, I went to the studio for some sessions.

The establishment of classes in Dundee came with some resistance. Opinions on yoga are usually based on prejudice. And the prejudice is that 'yoga is not for me', that 'meditation is not challenging enough' or that it is 'not physical enough'. I insist that it's really a fundamental practice in terms of exercise, physical and mental exercise for amputees, but also for people who have any kind of physical challenges.

To start with the term 'Yoga' – it comes from the Sanskrit and means to yoke together, union or connections. And to me, when you have an amputation, or a physical problem or injury, you lose contact with your body, with the connection with your body. And especially in the case of amputations and other major surgery, you need to literally redraw connections at all levels in your brain, in your mind, in your body.

I found that yoga for me was the pathway to get to know this new body and new me. To align, accept this new body and understand the limitations, but it is extraordinary what this new body can do. It's an empowering path. Because it allows you to realise it and acknowledge that yes, it's a different body, but it is not lesser.

Yoga encourages you to engage deeply with what is there, even absences. This is incredibly important to engage with, and it is empowering because you discover that, actually, you have an able body – more able than you or anyone else might think.

People tend to think that yoga is very easy and that it's not challenging enough. I think it's a really challenging practice, especially if you have any kind of physical disability or difficulty. And the challenge, for those who have never practised going inwards, is that it asks you to approach your body differently. It invites you to focus on all of you – body, mind and soul.

Yoga is for everybody, for every body. In my experience – pre and post amputation – I've done yoga when I had two legs, and I've done yoga with different teachers after my amputation, so I can make a comparison. I have experienced the different approaches that teachers take with their own practice, as well as their ideas and approaches to yoga. I have been in some classes with teachers whose idea is that there is one way of doing yoga and your body has to adapt and fit into that. But there are some poses that I am unable to do because of the mechanics of the prosthetic.

Whereas in other classes, like Finlay's, there is this ethos of learning together and exploring together – what works and what doesn't work for the whole class. The advantage is that the class I joined with Finlay is a class of everybody, with half of the class being amputees.

We are all very different. There are double amputees with no prosthetics. There are double amputees with prosthetics. Our prosthetics are really different and they do different things. It's not homogeneous. The best classes for me have always been classes where the teacher has admitted that they were learning with us. Because you might be an expert in yoga, but we are experts on disabled bodies.

Able or disabled bodies are unique. Finlay gives us options, because even if we are all amputees, some of us are maybe more mobile than others, or may enjoy being in the chair, standing or lying down more than others. With that, there is choice. There is collaboration.

Wholeness has little to do with the physical wholeness. In very practical terms, I would say that yoga is for everybody. I would say that there are no barriers other than the ones that oneself creates. Take the opportunity to begin a practice of alignment.

Dr Emilia Ferraro

After suffering amputations of my legs and hands following sepsis, I recognise how trauma affects the human body and how disabling that can be.

We all need different treatments, movements and therapies to help our bodies recover – one set style, position or pose doesn't fit all. Having someone who can ask, learn and understand the individual student before discussing the best treatments is vital, and we're delighted, at Finding Your Feet amputee charity, to have that in Finlay.

Our 'troopers' rave about him and what his work has done for their flexibility, movement and posture. Thanks for straightening us out, Finlay. I hope your book will allow lots more people to benefit from your experience. I'm a fan.

Cor Hutton, CEO Finding Your Feet

PART ONE

WHY CHAIR YOGA?

UNDERSTANDING THE FUNDAMENTALS OF AN ACCESSIBLE YOGA PRACTICE

CHAPTER ONE

INTRODUCTION

Anyone who has ever been to a yoga class has probably felt a tad confused, lost or intimidated by the experience. With so many styles of yoga, names of poses (that vary depending on who you ask), places and spaces used and the use or lack or props, there is a lot to take in if you have never been to a yoga class before. And that is before you even try a pose! That was certainly my experience.

I like to think that there is no bad time to start a yoga practice and no set way of doing things that renders energy expended futile. But I do wish I could go back and edit some parts of how I came to yoga as a practice and how I treated my body and mind in the early days. I've experienced so much learning and change that I would give to that younger practitioner and that influence the ways I deliver sessions now.

When I think about myself as a child and teenager/young person, I feel I wasn't conventionally sporty, but just because I wasn't involved in sports doesn't mean that I wasn't out walking, enjoying nature and learning about it. Physical activity wasn't something I set out to do deliberately, and yoga wasn't even in my view as an activity that was for me. I grew up in a small farming town in Scotland. I wasn't exposed to yoga growing up, and in the pre-internet days, the only reference materials I could have accessed would have been library books; yoga certainly didn't have my attention then. My interests lay in nature, music and history, but while my feet were on a specific path, I didn't know what lay ahead.

During my studies at the University of St Andrews, I was reading Classical Studies and Geography, but archaeology, environmental science and the way humans are affected by it captured my attention. I explored relationships with disease and the human body; rituals of healing, death and ceremony; and our changing relationships with the planet and ourselves. It is through this lens that I began to research human anatomy and sneak into the Medicine lecture halls, synthesising anatomy, literature, science and arts together. (Through the study of the ancient languages of Latin and Greek, I found comfort in the language of yoga and the language of anatomy. This only spurred me on to learn about and explore the use of Sanskrit, but that comes later.)

A few times in my teens I had difficulty with one of my legs, and when I was assessed by doctors it was put down to growing pains and I was told to get up and stretch my legs more often. During my second year at university, at 18, my condition had worsened, and I could no longer bend my left leg – after months and months of something grinding away and causing pain. Similar issues developed in my right leg, and I ended up having two corrective procedures on my legs six months apart, prolonging recovery and ultimately causing significant muscle loss. Along with nerve damage on my left leg, I had muscle loss and an invasive scar up to my right hip, which affected my movement. I spent nine months using mobility aids to get around, and unable to bear weight on my left leg without the knee buckling, I failed my motorbike compulsory basic training (CBT) test because I couldn't reliably take the weight of the vehicle on either leg. Added to this, emerging spinal problems in my lower back took me to regular physiotherapy appointments, where it was recommended I try yoga. At this point, yoga was not something on my radar – I had no real impression of what it would be like! Oh, to have had a trusty video to watch to prepare me...

My first experience of a yoga class was a few months post surgery. I arrived 45 minutes early in my crutches to speak with the instructor about the fact that I couldn't do any standing work but was still keen to learn. When the teacher did arrive, she looked me up and down and scoffed, saying, 'But we are doing standing work!' This moment shaped me, as I knew then that I wouldn't get help from this teacher and that I was being perceived as an inconvenience. I had very little access to other classes, being in a small town, and internet resources weren't great then either, so I stuck it out. We are talking pre-YouTube days, and social media had only just evolved to the point of having a poking feature on Facebook to make friends.

Starting a yoga practice can be daunting. We are asked to step into an unknown structure with rules, expectations and ethics while managing our own perceptions of what is going on. Personally, I find classes a real challenge, as group settings can be hard to navigate when you have specific considerations – be they related to injury, ability or learning type. When we are met with hostility, we make a shift internally to create a power dynamic that can feel a bit toxic, and for me, this meant I essentially bowed to the whims of the teacher without question.

What if we were welcomed with a smile and options were talked through? What if there was a resource to create a varied practice that would enable a practitioner to have the agency to engage in a class while skilfully modifying? What if someone's first class wasn't a comprehensive list of what they can't do but instead an exploration of all that they can do?

Being welcomed, encouraged and understood wasn't really my experience at all. I was in a world where physical ability and flexibility were celebrated, and any neediness or injury was treated as a nuisance. The system I was learning (even though I didn't even know it was a specific style at the time, as it was just called 'yoga') used a set sequence, the same poses every week with little to no variation. I was able to watch everyone do the first part of the class – standing poses, balances, etc. – and then I would join in the seated poses. I stuck with the class for six months, and then, while making a lot of notes, I started doing most of it at home. I used my home yoga practice in short bursts to alleviate pain while I was studying, and I even acquired some DVDs to try out different ways of moving. It was two years before my legs were reliable again, and while I was working a lot of sequences and poses, I still felt like I had something to prove in the previous system, and this is where I focused my energy. Over these two years, I would spend 20 minutes moving in the morning and another 20 minutes either in the evening or on a study break. I found that small, daily investment felt more beneficial to my body than one long session a week.

After graduating, I moved to Chicago and, not really knowing anyone there, I started attending some yoga classes. There was certainly a lot more on offer than in my small university town. I pushed hard into a system that looked for people to almost mark their proficiency by how far they could get in the poses (people would even ask what pose the person had gotten to in the sequence as a challenge in the changing room), and whenever I went to classes, part of me felt as if it could sustain all life if I was given praise, no matter how meagre, by the instructor. The system I was practising was very one-dimensional in the movement – a lot of forward bends, and it was with great earnestness that I pursued them. It was in this pursuit that my body had one more warning to give, and as I began learning to teach, my spine threw in the towel. I began to experience debilitating bouts of back pain, nerve dysfunction and loss of power in my legs that would plague me regularly beyond what I had experienced at the start of my yoga journey. It took over ten years to get a clear answer about what was wrong in my lower back, and there were a lot of hospital visits during these debilitating moments.

I am not sharing this with you to engender any kind of pity but more to express how these moments shaped my practice into what it is now. Each day when I get on my mat, I am looking to see what needs to move, what hurts and what I can do to guide my body to less pain. The ways I was treated in the yoga room, the bizarre rules that can exist in the yoga room, like not using props (even when you need them), and the way that we look at healing have all distilled into a way of working that feels totally different to the classes I attended. The structure of classes, the client intake process and even how pose variations are delivered is more compassionate and understanding, and as a teacher, it is much easier to create a sense of collaboration with these things in place.

The first classes I taught when I finished my teacher training were in a centre for adults with physical and learning disabilities. Every day was about variation and adaptability, with very little of what I learned in my teacher training being relevant (the training consisted of a lot of repetition of the Ashtanga Vinyasa sequence I mentioned – over and over again). I was initially trained in a set series, and this sequence is the same anywhere in the world – even the words and instructions are the same. The demands on the body are so rigorous that, even to this day, I haven't taught the full sequence to a single person. Some purists would demand that you do not use the name of their style of yoga if you even teach one pose differently or modify a pose for someone.

In 2011, a few years after I had moved to Dundee, having spent time training and completing my 500-hour teacher training modules, I knew I had to create a space for myself to teach. Working in gyms and community halls, I didn't have access to mats, props or really even a clean and quiet room in which to deliver sessions; it was time for a space of my own. Given the size of our city, there wasn't much else on the go except small pop-up classes, so I decided to take the leap into opening my own space, to set my own expectation levels and to provide the level of care and attention that was important to me.

I founded Heart Space Dundee, now Heart Space Yoga & Bodyworks, and in September 2011, after an intense period of renovations, we opened, with two studio spaces and two therapy rooms. Initially, we were offering beginner classes every day on a limited schedule with wide-ranging concessions; as a new organisation, we had to build up our reputation and confidence. We worked with organisations like Maggie's Centre Dundee, offering classes for people going through cancer treatments, and worked in schools with kids and young adults. We now have a team of 15 people delivering a diverse range of classes seven days a week – morning, afternoon and evening.

Using various tools of introspection, I have been able to look at my own values and start programmes with young people, kids and kids with additional support needs, which have now been running for over ten years, and our work has expanded to a full programme of free pre-natal, post-natal, kids and family classes that has brought our community together. Over the course of these ten years, we have worked with many clients of varying abilities, confident that we can create integrated class experiences that meet the needs of our community, regardless of economic status.

Since the pandemic, we have seen a reduction in services, with medical practices closing and appointments becoming digital, especially for physical injuries, and the number of people enquiring about more adaptable and accessible practices has increased dramatically. This led me to create a free chair yoga programme that would allow the charity to double up as a warm space, offering free tea before and after classes a few times a week. The sessions have been some of our most popular since our opening, and our plan is to continue to develop the programme; this is where this book comes in.

Over this period, I changed my teaching style from the rigours of the Ashtanga system as we began to see a greater swathe of the community, and adaptability became a moment-to-moment, pose-to-pose strategy, given the variability in the population. The diversity in our classes began to grow, especially around our use of props in classes and our expertise in chronic back conditions. My own experience as someone with numerous chronic injuries who had experienced debilitating periods of life, and 15 years' experience as a sports massage therapist, gave me great insight into the human body and how a practice can be negotiated to really fit the practitioner.

It was this direction towards injury resourcefulness and pose variation that drew me to Forrest Yoga. Never before had I encountered a system where there was an answer behind almost every 'why'. Anatomical information and innovation were at the core of the sequences, and props and variations were used in every session, regardless of the level of practitioner. Each session invited more connection and feeling rather than detachment and the pursuit of depth. The biggest difference was the use of intention to connect to a spot in the body and to investigate and negotiate with that area in a way that would inform the choices made in the class.

I would later come to realise that this focus work is a precursor to meditation on the yogic path.

Over the last few years at the yoga studio, we have seen a surge in interest in chair yoga, adaptive classes and sessions for amputees, and as we developed our curriculum, the resources seemed to be quite lacking, especially for people who wanted to practise at home. So, my reason for creating this book is twofold: to inspire teachers and movement professionals to be welcoming, well-versed and accommodating; and for practitioners to be inspired by how much they can do in their practice from a chair. As we work with more people, we see a rekindling. Not to distract from their efforts or to claim this as something we have done, but we see the revival of hope. We see a curiosity in navigating the body in a way that is really encouraging.

With a focus on posture, we can simplify our understanding of muscles – from over 600 muscles to a much more manageable 15, which are all responsible for spinal health. If we can create a practice that stimulates, lengthens and strengthens, then we will have a very full physical practice that allows for the effortless alignment of the bones. At the same time, yet this is seemingly separate, we will be navigating the nervous system through breathing techniques, building focus and meditation while also synthesising the ethics of a yoga practice like patience, acceptance and doing no harm. Combined, these weave together into a beautiful and nurturing system for healing.

The book is divided into themed exercise sections, including forward bends, back bends, twists and so on. I've included information about the benefits of each exercise alongside instructions for practice; this is to allow for a pose to be fully understood but also for instructors who may wish to share these practices with people and for practitioners. The information will be useful and makes up the 'why' part, but it won't be part of the pose experience each time; the pose cues will be the practical part to take away and consist of the 'doing' part. The poses come together with the sequences at the end of the book, and you may find yourself flipping back to a specific pose to refresh the main points. With familiarity comes ease!

Each chapter introduction has a little more information about the muscles we are targeting. It is my hope that you will treat this as optional, as sometimes the language of anatomy can feel quite daunting. When I lead training programmes, I like to focus on a smaller selection of muscles, so I invite you to have a read but worry less about integrating the information and focus more on the exercises in the chapter. Much like eating a sandwich, you don't need to know the makeup of each ingredient to know you are gaining something from it.

A NOTE ON LANGUAGE AND CUEING

For exercises that are upper body based, it is less important to focus on what the lower body is doing. I work with amputees, so I tend to avoid language about foot position unless the pose directly involves the feet. The primary focus should be on the body parts doing the pose; the rest is along for the ride.

CHAPTER TWO

THE FUNDAMENTALS

STRUCTURING YOUR PRACTICE

When I structure my own practice, very seldom do I do the same thing all the time. As I mentioned, I explore the needs of the body each day, but while you are new to the practice, it can be good to choose variety. Our day-to-day lives, especially if they are more sedate, involve a lot of the same movements. How often do you have your arms over your head each day? Adding variety of movement allows a diversification from repetitive sedentary postures to full body articulation. I like clients I work with to rotate movement themes. For example, if on Monday we primarily do forward bends, then the next day we would do something different, maybe twists or back bends. Or, if I had a day where I was sitting a lot, I might do a bit of lower body or hip work. I hope that through seeing and experiencing a large vocabulary of poses, you are genuinely inspired to practise whatever you feel you need, and with practice, you will become more skilful at knowing what your body needs.

When creating a sequence for yourself, sometimes you just need one or two poses to hit the spot, but if you are looking to do a longer practice, some sequencing observations can be really helpful. When creating a longer practice, taking time to set an intention for the session brings a very different quality of attention. This is a very empowering action, allowing the practitioner to track sensation changes and make decisions based on the set intention.

Warming up the joints, especially if you are planning any weight bearing, is essential at the start of the practice, not just to get the joints lubed up but also to build the mental representations of the muscles before more significant demands are made of them. I also like to add in smaller versions of movements that will be done later. After warming up, more dynamic movements that demand more strength can be done safely, building on the foundations of the warm-up. After that, warming down and cooling down can help bring the body closer to a more restful and integrative state. It is this format that will allow your practice to feel rewarding and enriching in its variety and adaptability.

In a 60-minute format, that would look like:

2 minutes: Intent setting

23 minutes: Warm-up

20 minutes: Hot part (where we really get moving)

10 minutes: Warm-down

5 minutes: Cool-down

Following this roughly, even for a shorter practice, means you can create wonderful sequences that feel intelligent and engage with the body in a way that can create postural change.

Intent Setting and Examples

Setting an intent is not about creating an end result but a way to build focus in your practice. Choosing something tangible that you can feel and track is more important than choosing something global or cosmic. Here are some of my favourite intentions to work with:

- 'What do I need today? Is there a specific part of my body that needs this class the most today?'

- 'Pick an area for healing. Work in a way that brings space and relief into that spot for the entire practice.'

- 'Breathe in a soothing way in every pose.'

- 'Feel the vitality in your own body. Do this by bringing attention into the visceral sensations of each pose.'

Warm-up: Includes pranayama (breathwork), mobilisation, joint lubrication, resistance drills and movement of injury or tweaky areas. The warm-up should give consideration to what joints will be impacted during the class and warmed up to get the synovial fluid circulating.

Hot part: Includes core work, dynamic movement, weight bearing and deeper poses. A lot of yoga systems relegate core work to the end of a class or begin with sun salutations to warm up, but in my experience, getting the core fired up at the start not only helps with deep breathing but also gets the body ready for bigger movements. It is in this section that poses usually adhere to a theme – if we are doing twists, we will build into gradually bigger twisting movements in this section before warming down.

Warm-down: Unwind poses that are less strenuous versions of poses in the hot part, with longer holds. Ending a session with the muscles feeling long, relaxed and at ease is a great way to enter into relaxation. Taking rest with the muscles feeling strained from work can just make everything a bit uncomfortable. It is important to take the time to bring the body down from the excitement and upregulation of the hot part.

Cool-down: This is a time for relaxation, breathwork or meditation to assist integration of all the postural work in the session. A position that is comfortable, where no stretch or strain is on the body, is best. It can take time to develop an affinity for this section, but with practice and support, it can be the most rewarding.

PROPS AND EQUIPMENT

For the practices in this book, a chair is really all that you need. A sturdy and firm chair, ideally without armrests, gives a little more room for movement, but so long as the chair won't tip over easily, then it will work. I recommend working with a yoga mat under the chair to stop any slipping and to provide support when contacting the ground. As you progress through the book, you will meet poses that use one or more block and a strap. These standard yoga tools are easy to find and are relatively inexpensive (they can even be found in most supermarkets). They allow us to have more options when we need a bit more support, and if there is a takeaway message from this book, it is to take support when you can get it! In place of a strap, a towel or dressing gown cord could easily be used. Some poses also use a bolster, which is a sturdy cushion, but a bed pillow can be used instead. Again, it creates a support that is useful for variation. I also use a rolled-up yoga mat (folded into thirds and rolled up, and a towel would work too) and a blanket to create different resistance from squeezing a block. If you are a yoga teacher,

I think it is good to have these things, even if you personally don't use them, so they can be available for those who do need them.

> Since coming to chair classes, my limitations have really opened up. I find I'm twisting a lot easier, a lot better. I'm getting that extra few millimetres. I feel my movement in general is much more fluid, much more supple.
>
> I do small movements, small poses in bed at night using poses from class. So, 20 minutes to 30 minutes at night before I go to sleep, I find that I get a sleep right through the night.
>
> This time last year, even before I got my second surgery, I wouldn't have been able to do that...
>
> If I stretch cleaning the windows or do the hoovering, I want to not feel sore afterwards. So since I came out of the hospital in September and got my second limb and started coming to chair classes, I personally, mentally, physically and emotionally have evolved.

Scott

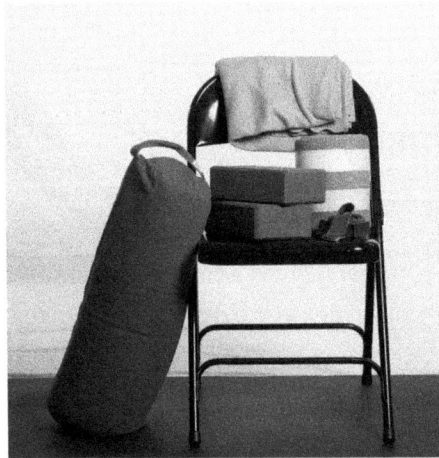

BASIC MOVES

In each pose, there could be an exhaustive list of the various ways to move and engagements to feel for, but in the system I teach, some basics can be observed and implemented really well. In some instances, you may find yourself working all of the basic moves at the same time.

 'Basic' can be misinterpreted as 'Beginner' or 'Not for Advanced People', but these basic moves are for every level – beginner, intermediate, advanced. Consider that 'Basic' means 'Foundation'. For anything to exist and thrive, it needs a foundation. Basic moves provide helpful support so that change is doable and much easier. The basic moves break habitual patterns of being in the body and bring into focus the mind-body connection.

Active feet: To develop conscious connection, active feet is an important action in many poses to maintain a strong quality of attention. Not only does this create a grounding and stabilising action in most poses, but the activation also strengthens muscles in the feet and lower legs that provide support to the knees. To switch this on, press into the heels with about 70% of the weight, and with the remaining 30%, press into the base of the toes and lift and spread the toes from the big toe to the pinkie toe. Even if there is no visually evident spread, keep this activation. There are very few exceptions to using active feet, except during rest and relaxation poses.

Active hands: We spend so much of our time holding phones, computers, TV remotes, walking sticks, etc., and the hands, wrists and forearms can be a surprising place of tension and discomfort in the body. To work active hands, the aim is to spread from the pinkie finger to the thumb, energise the fingers and spread the palm with the wrist joint kept neutral. In seated poses, this should invigorate the forearms to the elbow so that when we bear weight in the hands, they are resilient and strong.

Tuck the tailbone: There are some poses where tucking the pelvis downwards will allow for activation in the lower abdominal muscles. This is the primary physical action in our core work and in poses like bridge. Usually, it is used in standing poses in conjunction with telescoping the ribs up. The primary aim is to decompress the lower back. Every person has a variable presentation of a neutral pelvis and lower back curvature, so some people may need to do more movement with this and some less. When combined with the following technique, they balance one another out using the core to provide support.

Telescope the ribs: This sensation consists of moving the ribs away from the pelvis, mid ribs away from the lower ribs and upper ribs away the from mid ribs, and also moving the back ribs up. Sometimes this sensation of lengthening can feel easier than mentioning spinal length. Similar to the previous technique, different poses require varying amounts of application. In some of the poses, you will see a hand placed on the skull to give a prompt to lengthen the spine and telescope the ribs up/forwards, etc.

Relaxed neck: This is one of the more noticeable differences in my classes. Many systems encourage gaze points (drishti) beyond, or to the hand or to the foot. In my experience, when there are any postural issues in the upper back or neck, these positions can kink the neck and cause injury. As many of the poses in this book are supported, and there is ample neck work to develop a healthy relationship with the postural muscles, the aim is to work in all poses with a relaxed neck. Rather than totally flopping the neck, the priority is to feel that there is no neck strain as a result of the poses. In poses where we are deliberately stretching the neck, we are still looking to be without strain and for the stretch to be around a 6 on a comfort scale (with 1 being no stretch and 10 being excruciating).

Wrap the shoulders: This technique begins as a spreading of the shoulder blades, and in poses like side bends, refers to both the rotation of the arm and shoulder blade and the lifting of the arm. Many people in classes or on the massage table hold a lot of tension here and frequently have issues with moving the shoulder blades freely on the ribs. With a focus on shoulder mobility in this book, the action of wrapping the shoulder blades and spreading them wide may feel challenging, but I recommend developing familiarity with the move 'unlocking the shoulder' (see Chapter Three) to get a feel for the movement potential you can unlock there. This technique can then be used in many of the poses.

Deep breathing: Chapter Eleven will explore breathwork in more detail. Throughout the sessions and poses, I encourage you to feel for a full diaphragmatic breath. Aim to feel the abdomen moving on an inhale for a slow count of five and engaging inwards on an exhale for a slow count of six. This inhale for five and exhale for six format is what we use in all poses unless otherwise specified. Abdominal breathing allows for pressure changes to be felt in the abdomen and chest cavity, increased flexibility of the entire ribcage, recruitment of muscles of inspiration (that sounds inspiring!) and the dissociation of hiking the shoulders up with each inhalation.

Each of the sample classes will also work with specific breathing exercises at the start, but the prevailing breath form during a session would be deep ujjayi breathing.

PART TWO

PRACTICES

CHAPTER THREE

WARMING UP

For a practice that will last a lifetime, don't overlook warming up! Many systems of movement can be a bit light on the warm-up section of a class, jumping straight into complex multi-faceted movement or assuming that the practitioner may have warmed themselves up beforehand. In a yoga class setting, unless the movement themes have been announced previously, people can't be expected to know which muscles they should warm up. They can move their own achier parts and areas that need extra attention, but I think the responsibility is on the teacher to create an engaging warm-up that feels like part of the main body sequencing of the class (the hot part).

This section will take you through many different movements and static poses that you can include in a warm-up. When looking at the theme of a class (i.e., whether the focus is on twisting, weight bearing on the hands, back bending, etc.) it is useful to look at the poses as if they have nutritional qualities, much like preparing a meal. We want to prepare our spice mixes and ingredients ahead of time before we bring it all together, and intelligent class planning is just like that. If, for example, we are building back bends towards camel with a strap, it would be a good idea to explore some spinal articulation, like cat arches, and some shoulder mobilisation to complement what will be demanded of the body later. This may mean that your warm-up section looks different each day. Alternatively, you may find that some of the poses and exercises in this section become daily staples for you, regardless of what the theme of the class is. Personally, I find that the neck isometric work feels great when my neck and shoulders ache even if the theme doesn't involve the shoulders and neck.

Fundamental to the warm-up experience is the time taken for pre-assessment, mobilisation, connection and engagement. Pre-assessment, a simple check-in with one's own body, before arriving at more complicated poses allows you to connect with how the body is feeling and moving each day, and identify areas of specific need, injury areas, or places that you want to focus your attention on. This is a rewarding part of the process, and it is prudent to avoid injuries from practice (even the best intentions in the world and the best planning can't prevent injury, but we can set ourselves up for success).

Mobilisation allows an exploration of the moving joints in isolation, moving through full ranges of motion and articulating individual body parts. When we start to map out practices by theme, your understanding of what to mobilise will increase and become more skilful. As you develop experience, you will know what feels really good when preparing for back bends versus what feels good when warming up for forward bends. These smaller movements and articulations help prepare both the body and the mind for what is going to happen next, allowing for a sense of ease and calm when similar, perhaps more challenging movements are met later in the sequence. For example, if I am going into a big twisting forward bend, and I've moved my spine, gently twisted and navigated spinal articulation, I will be in a better place to feel whether I need props for a pose and the movement pathways that need to be explored. This process of movement mapping is a great way to take the fear out of poses and create a steady and relaxed environment while practising.

Here are a couple more examples:

Apex Pose: Twisting Warrior

This pose involves the hips, hip flexors, spine, core and shoulders.

Warm-up suggestions: Shoulder shrugs, shoulder flossing with a strap, stage 3, seated side bend, hip mobility twist, twist.

Apex Pose: Pyramid

This is a big forward bend that involves the hamstrings, lower back and hips.

Warm-up suggestions: Quad extensions, cat, adductor and abductor isolations, block step overs.

Some of this movement mapping may take the form of smaller versions of the poses, longer holds, muscle activations and repetitions that engage both fast- and slow-twitch muscles fibres through different movement qualities. Some of the poses in this section are made up of breath-to-movement elements where you are moving dynamically and others where you are static, and these will be clearly labelled. Not to confuse things, but some of the warm-up exercises are absolute gold – you may find that bringing a set of them back in later would work well. Sometimes my hamstrings take a while to negotiate, so I revisit the same warm-up again later in the hot part to check in with how they are getting on.

WRIST STRETCHES – FINGER PULLS

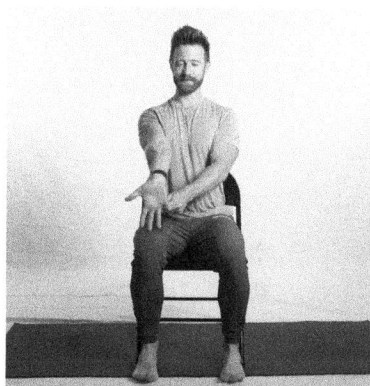

The wrists take a lot of strain in our day-to-day lives, and the default is for the fingers to curl in towards the palm. These individual finger pulls can help stretch not only the palm but also the muscles on the underside of the forearm – the wrist flexors.

► Extend the left palm forwards with the fingers pointing down, taking care that the elbow isn't locked.

► Inhale, take a hold of the pinkie finger of the left hand with the right fingers.

► Exhale, pull back on the pinkie and spread the fingers and palm wide.

► Repeat a full breath cycle for each finger and then do the other hand. One pull per finger is enough.

WRIST EXTENSOR STRETCH – POUR

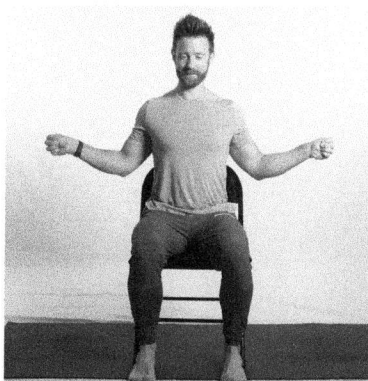

Continuing our circumnavigation of wrist tension, the pour can be very useful to alleviate tight and movement limited wrists.

► Inhale to fully open the palms with the arms out to the sides with the elbows in a relaxed bend. The thumbs point up and palms face forwards.

► Exhale to fold the thumbs in first, curl all

the fingers around the thumbs and make an action as if pouring from a jug – a downward movement on the wrist, keeping the closed palm facing forwards – while squeezing the thumbs about 50%.

▶ Repeat this one more time.

WRIST EXTENSOR STRETCH – CURL

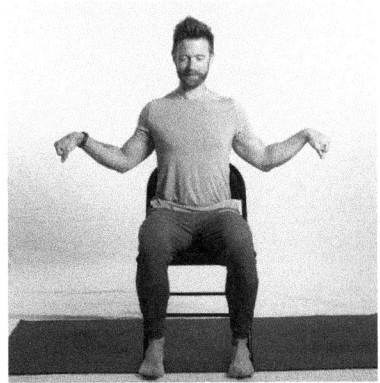

This time, we are stretching the wrist extensors, which are usually quite tight.

▶ Open the arms out to the sides with the elbows in a relaxed bend.

▶ Inhale to open the palms with the palms facing down.

▶ Exhale to curl the fingers in, with the thumbs on the outside of the fingers this time, and draw the knuckles down towards the floor. Do a 50% squeeze (or whatever your tolerance level is for this).

▶ Repeat this one more time.

CAT

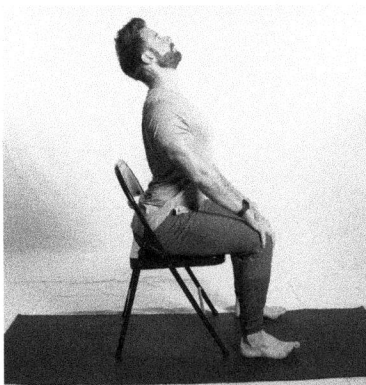
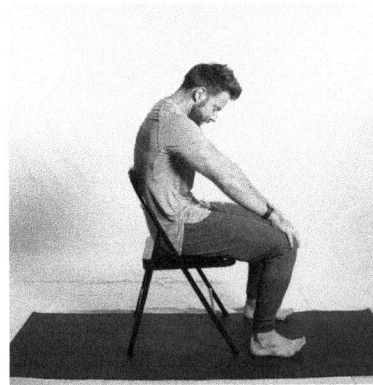

These two seated cat exercises should be on your list to do every day to create movement in your spine. There will be sections that feel more mobile and areas that may feel a bit stuck. Our aim is to gently move and articulate each area. There are two strategies we can use here: move from the central spine or try to move each section of the spine in order, from the pelvis to the skull.

Cat – Extension

▶ Inhale, scoop the chest forwards, lift the skull and stick your butt out.

Cat – Flexion

▶ Exhale, round the chest forwards, tuck the tailbone under and allow the head to come forwards.

▶ Repeat for eight rounds of both the inhale and exhale movements.

▶ You can add an extra detail to this by drawing the shoulder blades together on the inhale to assist in the chest moving forwards. On the exhale, spread the shoulder blades to get more rounding into the upper thoracic spine.

CAT VARIATIONS

Shoulder Blade Squeeze

This cat variation allows for extra movement of the shoulder joints and upper back. It is particularly helpful for anyone who struggles with shoulder blade wrapping or is looking to thoroughly warm up the shoulders. As with the previous cat exercise, these two poses are linked by breath.

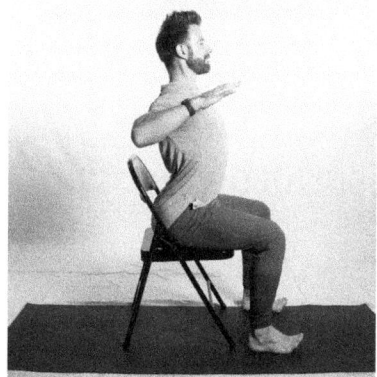

▶ Note that the spinal breath action is reversed to assist the movement of the shoulders.

▶ Exhale to squeeze the shoulder blades together with the arms bending and parallel to the ground.

Shoulder Blade Spread

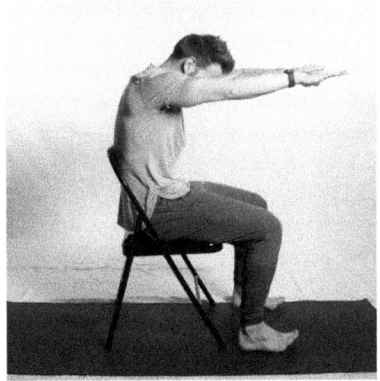

- ▶ Inhale to round into the upper back, arms raised and reaching forwards, and spreading the shoulder blades wide.

- ▶ Repeat this with the previous cat variation eight times.

BOW PULLS

This shoulder warm-up allows for each shoulder blade to explore independent movement, a physical action that can be quite stuck.

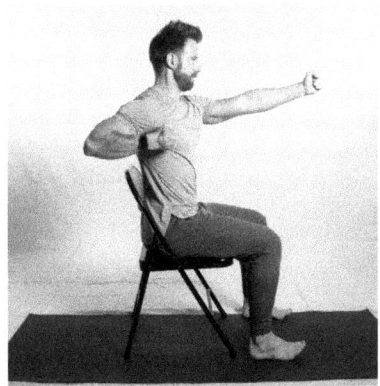

- ▶ Start with both arms raised forwards and shoulder distance apart.

- ▶ Exhale to pull back the right arm as if pulling back on a bow. Squeeze the right shoulder blade back and reach the left arm and shoulder blade forwards.

- ▶ Inhale to return to the start position and then repeat on the other side.

- ▶ Repeat six times on each arm.

SHOULDER FLOSSING

Start Position

The stages in this shoulder-flossing series can either be done together or split up. It creates a great range of motion for the shoulders, upper back and thoracic spine, which enables many different movements. This can be performed with the arms at shoulder distance apart or slightly wider apart, with a strap or a towel.

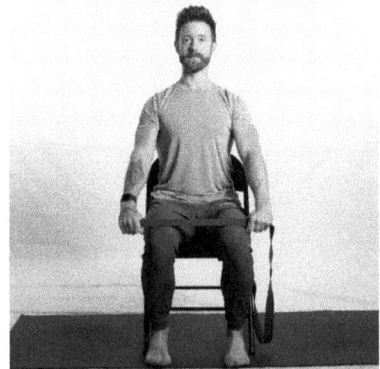

For each stage, the start position is arms down but with an active pulling action outwards.

Shoulder Flossing: Stage 1

▶ Beginning in the start position, create a slight external rotation (so the elbows face forwards) of the upper arms while pulling outwards on the strap.

▶ Inhale to lift the arms overhead maintaining tension on the strap.

▶ Exhale to lower the strap down to the start position.

▶ Repeat ten times.

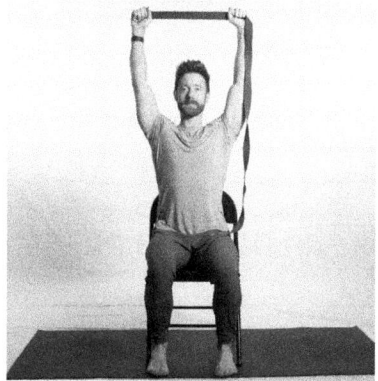

Shoulder Flossing: Stage 2

▶ Beginning in the start position, inhale to lift the arms up through stage 1.

▶ Exhale to twist the chest to the left with tension in the strap keeping the shoulders level.

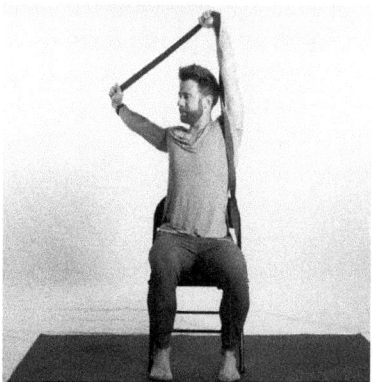

▶ Inhale back to seated with the arms up.

▶ Exhale to return to the start position.

▶ Repeat on the other side and then repeat fully four more times.

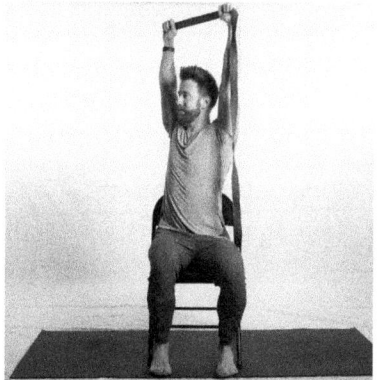

Shoulder Flossing: Stage 3

▶ Beginning in the start position, inhale to lift the arms up through stage 1.

▶ Exhale to twist the chest to the left with tension in the strap, keeping the shoulders level.

▶ Pull down on the left arm and reach up with the right arm keeping both arms straight.

▶ Inhale back to seated with the arms up.

▶ Exhale to return to the start position.

▶ Repeat on the other side and then repeat fully four more times.

REAR DELTOID PRESS

The rear deltoid is often quite a weak muscle, and even in experienced practitioners, it can easily be overlooked.

▶ Holding the strap with both hands behind the back and chair, lift the arms away from the back at a 45-degree angle.

▶ Inhale to lift the chest.

▶ Exhale to press back with the hands, drawing outwards on the strap with the arms lifting towards parallel to the ground. Hold for eight breaths.

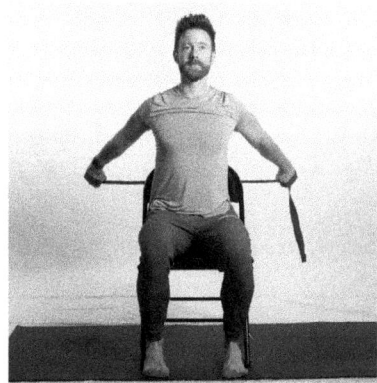

NECK ISOMETRICS

Isometric actions build muscle tone and awareness that supports the various postural muscles in the neck. The aim of this exercise is to feel muscles switching on rather than to create movement.

Work three breath cycles on the front of the head, both sides of the head and the back of the head.

Neck Isometrics – Front

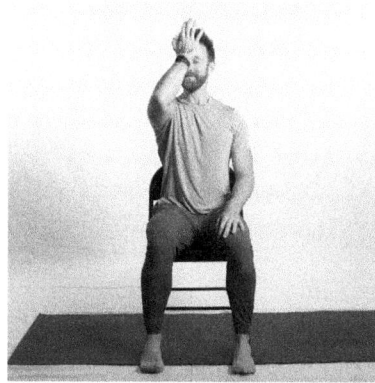

- ▶ Inhale in an upright position with the head and neck tall.

- ▶ Raise one hand and place it on the forehead.

- ▶ Exhale to press the head into the hand to create tension in the muscles.

- ▶ Inhale to release the pressure. Repeat three times.

Neck Isometrics – Rear

This technique is also useful to prepare for twists or anytime that you are unsure of your head and neck position being neutral.

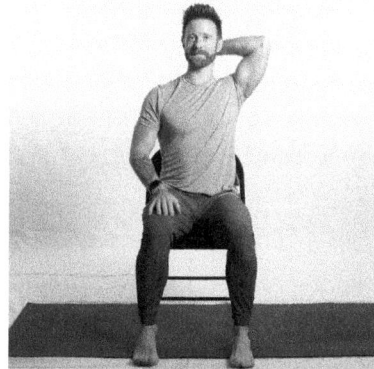

- ▶ Raise one hand and place it on the back of the head.

- ▶ Inhale in an upright position with the head and neck tall.

- ▶ Exhale to press the head into the hand to create tension in the muscles.

- ▶ Inhale to release the pressure.

- ▶ Repeat three times before moving to another part of the head and neck.

Neck Isometrics – Sides

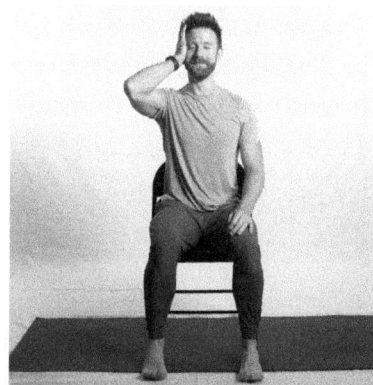

- ▶ Raise a hand and place it on the side of the head.

- ▶ Inhale in an upright position with the head and neck tall.

- ▶ Exhale to press the head into the hand to create tension in the muscles.

- ▶ Inhale to release the pressure.

- ▶ Repeat three times before swapping sides.

NECK ROTATIONS

Working neck rotation into regular practice can be very useful for improving the posture of the upper body. Neck tension contributes to shoulder pain, nerve issues in the arms and hands, headaches and chronic tension in the upper body.

During the repetitions, maintain the head level so it doesn't become a side bend, especially at the end of the range of motion.

▶ Inhale to telescope the ribs and spine up.

▶ Exhale to rotate the head to the left until you can't move it any further.

▶ Inhale back to centre.

▶ Repeat on the other side.

▶ Repeat for six more rounds.

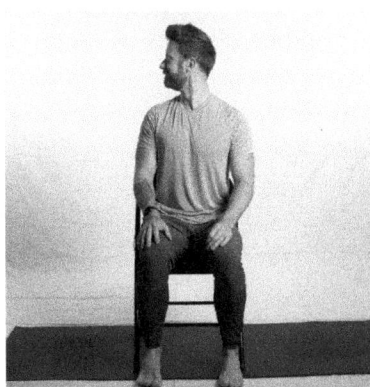

SHOULDER SHRUGS

This movement should be a daily staple of practice. Splitting the shoulder blades into three parts, the aim is to feel movement in the top, middle and lower parts of the shoulder blades. With each lower section, there is less potential movement, so do not be discouraged about that. This is a wonderful posture builder for the trapezius, rhomboids and latissimus dorsi muscles.

▶ Inhale to spread the shoulders wide with the arms relaxed by your side. Hold the breath, shrug the shoulders up by the ears. Exhale to squeeze the shoulders back and drag them down.

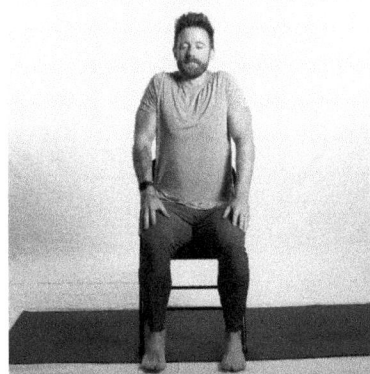

▶ Inhale to spread the shoulders wide; exhale to squeeze them straight back and down.

▶ Inhale to spread the upper back and turn the palms to face up with the elbows bent, exhale to squeeze the bottom part of the blades towards each other and drag down.

ACTIVE ARCHER

Full archer is usually quite passive when the hands meet, but I find that to develop strength and familiarity of this movement pathway, you have to build this pattern.

▶ For active archer, reach one arm up and one arm down. The shoulder of the raised arm is wrapping forwards; the lower arm is pressing back to feel the rear deltoid.

▶ Inhale to telescope the ribs up.

▶ Exhale to press both hands backwards as if you were pushing them into a wall behind you, without the chest flaring into a back bend.

▶ Hold for eight breaths, take a small break and then work the other side.

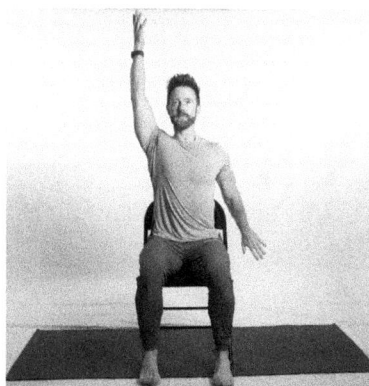

EAGLE ARMS PREPARATION

We will encounter eagle arms later, but this is a great way to both move the shoulder blades and strengthen the chest muscles for this adduction.

▶ Slip the strap behind the back, just underneath the shoulder blades, and hold the ends in front of you. The strap should be under the arms and held firmly in the hands, with the elbows bent roughly 90 degrees.

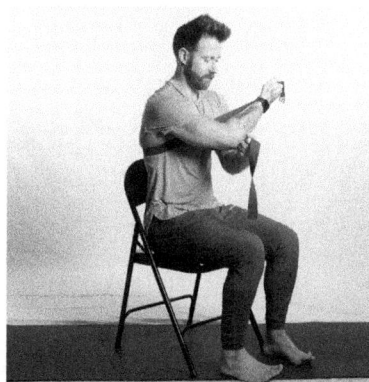

▶ Inhale to hold the straps forwards and parallel.

▶ Exhale to cross the arms at the elbows as best as you can while flexing the chest muscles.

▶ Inhale to return to centre. Repeat on the other side and cross the other arm on top. Repeat six times.

EAGLE ARMS ROTATIONS

Building on the chest activation of the previous exercise, these circles can create small movements of the shoulder joint towards larger movement of the entire upper back section and ribs, which can be very tight and restricted.

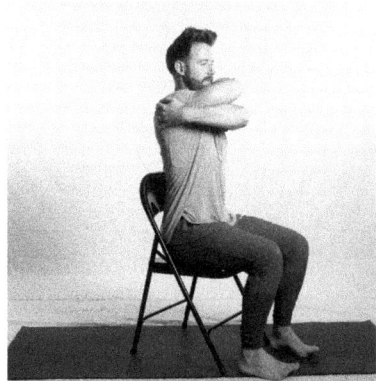

▶ Leave a bit of space between the back and the chair and cross the left arm over the right arm like a self-hug, with the hands resting on the shoulders. The fingers pull on the shoulder or upper arm to walk the arms into a tighter wrap. Use the fingers to help draw the elbows towards being stacked.

▶ Begin to make small circles with the arms, keeping the torso and neck completely still. Do three circles and then reverse the direction.

▶ Repeat on the other side with the right arm on top of the left.

▶ Come back to the original side, make larger circles that point the elbows upwards and then in a circular action, allowing the ribcage to move with the arms. Make three big thoracic circles – as large as you can make them – and reverse the directions. Repeat on the other side.

EAGLE ARMS

Once the shoulders are a little more warmed up, this pose can access some of the sticky places in the upper back. Eagle arms encourages the shoulder blades to spread on the back, assisting with the assimilation of the basic move or wrapping the shoulder blades. Be aware that there will be some pressure on the wrist extensors of the forearm. If the wrap of the hands isn't yet doable, the option of holding the upper outer arms, as used in the eagle arms rotations, works well.

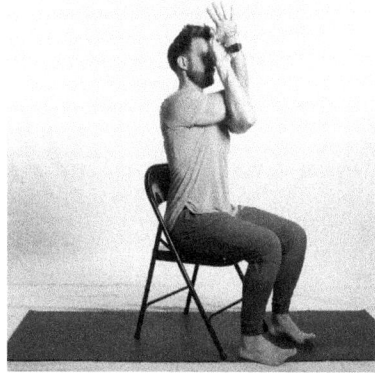

▶ Leave a bit of space between the back and the chair and cross the left arm over the right arm with the elbows bent and the upper arms parallel to the floor. Aim to get the forearms perpendicular to the ground.

▶ Bring the right hand closer to your face and hold the thumb of the left hand.

▶ Hold for eight breaths and repeat on the other side.

KITE HAWK

Kite Hawk Internal Rotation

This is a dynamic rotation exercise. It involves moving the arms and shoulders into internal rotation in this part of the practice and external rotation in the next part of the practice. Kite hawk also moves the upper spine, so you will experience a bit of movement in the head and neck.

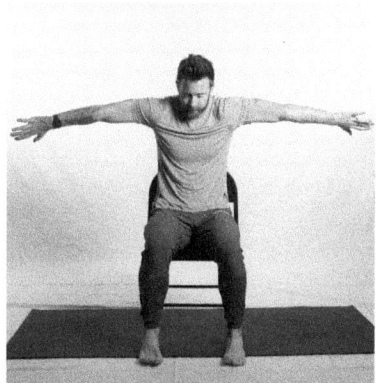

▶ Start with the arms out to the side, level with the shoulders.

▶ Exhale to internally rotate the arms without dropping them, allowing the upper back and neck to round forwards slightly.

Kite Hawk External Rotation

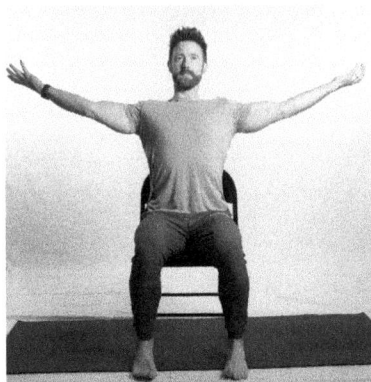

▶ Inhale to rotate the palms to face up, exploring the external rotation of both arms. This will create a slight lift in the chest and neck area.

▶ Repeat the internal and external rotations eight more times.

▶ This should feel smooth and easy; if it hurts, reduce the range of motion.

Kite Hawk Alternating

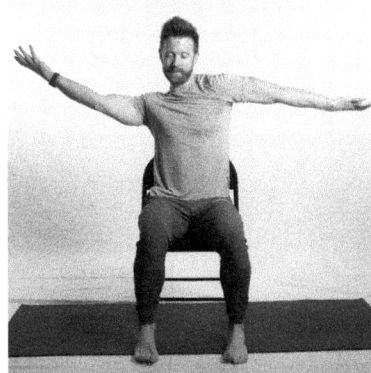

There is a lot to be said for movement patterns that ask one side of the body to move counter to the other. This movement allows for the upper back and chest to very slightly twist as the arms explore the internal and external rotations of kite hawk.

▶ Inhale to sit with the arms out to the side and level with the shoulders and palms facing forwards.

▶ Exhale to internally rotate one arm and externally rotate the other. The chest will twist very slightly.

▶ Repeat eight more times.

DYNAMIC THORACIC TWISTS

A lot of folks tend to move the lower back and neck during twists, with very little movement around the mid and upper back – the thoracic spine. This can be used to warm up straight before a static twist.

In this exercise, the pelvis stays still by pressing down into the feet.

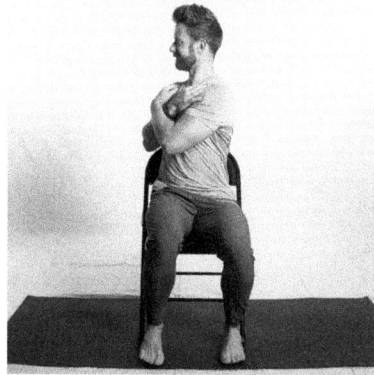

▶ Cross the arms on the chest (or place them behind the head for extra postural demand).

▶ Inhale to telescope the ribs up and press into active feet.

▶ Exhale to rotate to the right without moving the pelvis or rotating the neck, spine long.

▶ Inhale back to centre and repeat six more times before swapping to the other side.

BRIDGE WITH A ROLL

If bridge on the floor isn't possible, this is a great way to create a similar action in the lower body, a bit of spinal extension, chest opening and inner thigh activation.

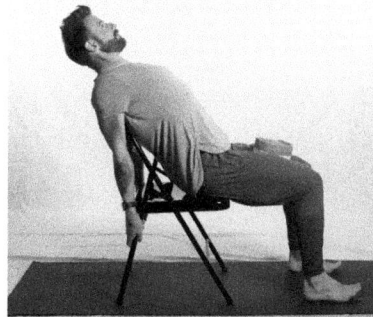

▶ Slide towards the front of the seat and lean the upper body against the rear rest of the chair – you may need to pad it with a blanket. Place a roll (a rolled up mat or towel) or block between the thighs.

▶ Inhale to telescope the ribs up.

▶ Exhale, press into active feet, squeeze the inner thighs on the roll and reach the arms down the sides of the chair. Depending on the chair, you may be able to reach the rear legs.

▶ Hold here for ten breaths.

SIDE BEND WITH NECK RELEASE

Seated side bend and neck release are frequently linked together and are a great way to warm up the wrapping of the shoulders, create a sense of space in the lower back and reconfigure the upper back and neck.

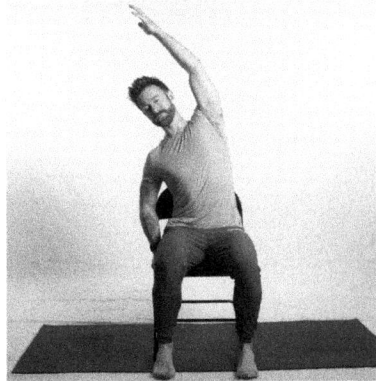

▶ Brace one hand onto the hip or frame of the chair.

▶ Inhale to lift the opposite arm up overhead.

▶ Exhale to wrap the lifted arm's shoulder blade forwards and lean into the side bend.

▶ Stay here for eight breaths before moving the top arm down towards neck release (the next practice).

NECK RELEASE (FOLLOWING ON FROM SIDE BEND)

▶ From your seated side bend, exhale to move the top arm until the hand is lower than the shoulder.

▶ Inhale to telescope the ribs up, creating space in the lower back.

▶ Exhale to roll both shoulder blades down.

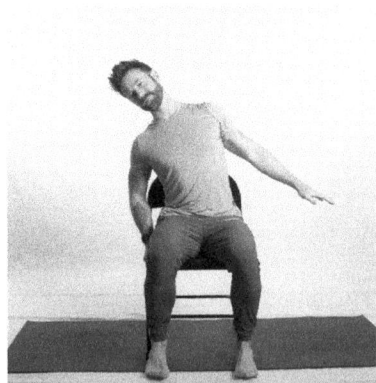

▶ For tension in the trapezius, tilt the chin down but not the entire head; for a tight chest/collarbone area, tilt the chin up.

▶ Hold for eight breaths before coming back up with your neck relaxed. Use the arm that was supporting on the chair to lift the head back to the start position.

DYNAMIC HIP MOBILITY TWIST

Moving the hip joints, especially if one is sitting a lot, is really important. Even in a diverse yoga practice, the action of internally rotating the thigh is seldom navigated.

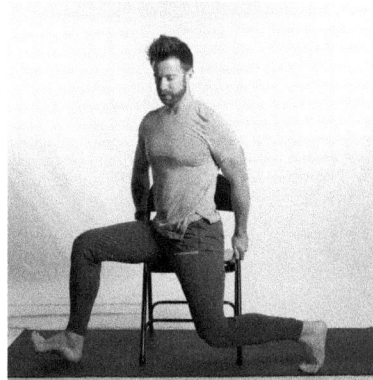

▶ Starting in a seated position with the legs wide, inhale to lift the spine up.

▶ Exhale to turn the left leg to the left and the right leg to the left at roughly 90-degree angles so that the right knee points downwards.

▶ Inhale back to centre. Exhale to repeat, sending the right leg to the right and the left leg to the right.

▶ Repeat this six times each side, alternating sides.

DYNAMIC BLOCK STEP OVERS

Tight muscles are seldom strong muscles. They have been robbed of their ability to lengthen and contract, so while it may seem counter-intuitive to build strength in these areas, it can revolutionise their function. Block step overs get the hip flexors, adductors and abductors engaging and developing awareness. For more of a challenge, the blocks can be set increasingly higher or the stepping onto the block stage can even be missed out by going right over the top.

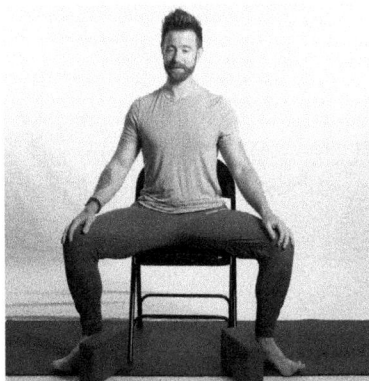

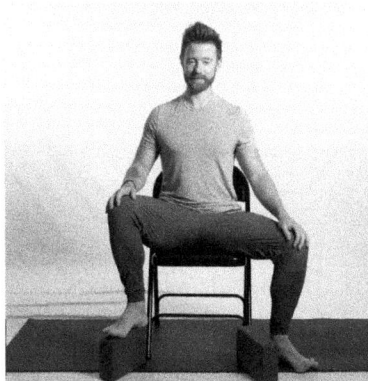

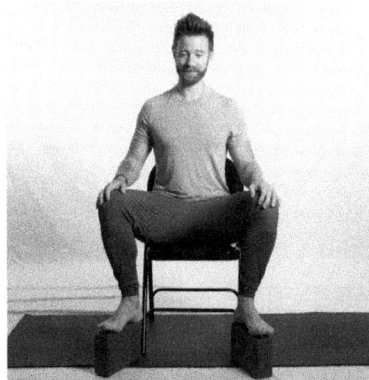

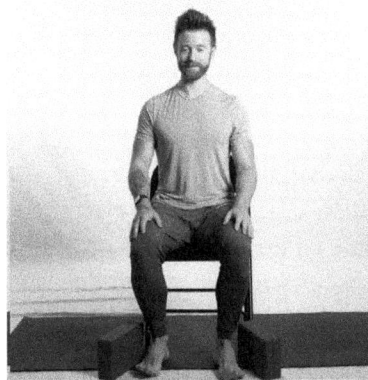

- ▶ Start with the feet wider than hip distance apart and place two blocks on the floor to the insides of the ankles.

- ▶ Exhale to step the left foot onto the left block and then the right foot onto the right block.

- ▶ Inhale to step the feet down to the insides of the block – first left and then right.

- ▶ Exhale to step the right foot out onto the block followed by the left.

- ▶ Inhale to step the feet down to the outside of the block – right and then left.

- ▶ Repeat this six more times, alternating the leading leg.

DYNAMIC QUAD EXTENSIONS

This is a set-up for stretching the hamstrings, flexing the hip and exploring the relationship with the lower back. This practice is the inhale portion of the exercise, and the part below ('Dynamic Quad Extensions (Extension)') is the exhale portion.

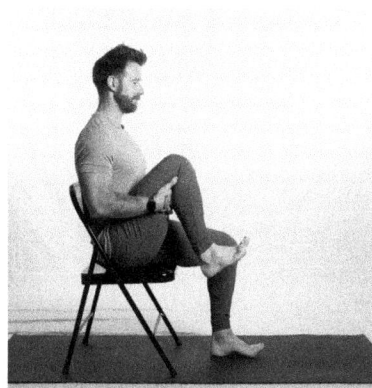

▶ With the back against the frame of the chair, draw one thigh into your chest, aiming to get it as close to the chest as possible without the lower back rounding.

Dynamic Quad Extensions (Extension)

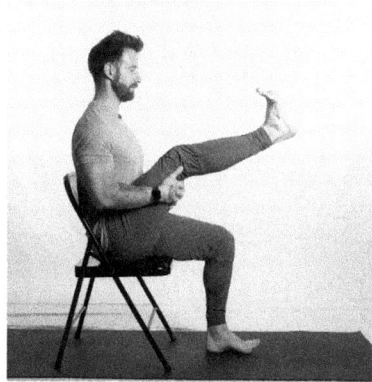

▶ Exhale and attempt to straighten the leg; it is unlikely to straighten fully, but you will feel your thighs engage and hamstrings lengthen.

▶ With the exertion, aim to lift the spine and keep the pelvis still.

▶ Inhale to bend the leg, bracing the thigh against the chest.

▶ Repeat the leg extension ten times and hold the last round for eight breaths.

▶ Repeat six more times and then change legs.

ANKLE ROTATIONS AND POINT AND FLEX

When exploring poses where the feet are on the floor for support or for balance, exploring the movement range of the ankle is important. By increasing circulation and moving lethargic muscles, you can warm up all the muscles that support the lower leg and knee.

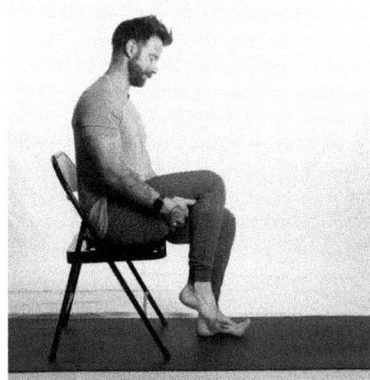

► Either hold the thigh to raise the foot or lift the foot off the floor and begin to make rotations of the foot in a smooth and steady action.

► Do eight rotations and then repeat in the other direction.

► After the rotations, begin to flex and point the foot, moving smoothly through your comfortable range of motion.

► Flex and point eight times and repeat fully on the other side.

DOUBLE QUAD EXTENSIONS

Warming up the quads to straighten the legs can simultaneously stretch the backs of the legs and build strength in the fronts of the leg, supporting the knee joints. Bracing the arms on the chair also makes this a pose that will engage your core muscles and hip flexors.

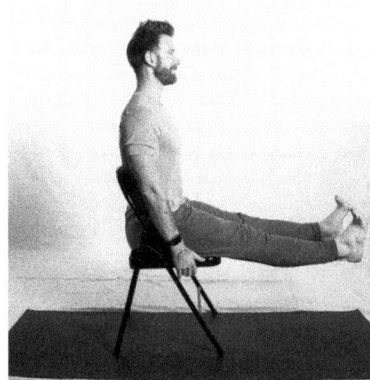

► Bracing the hands on the chair frame, sit back against the backrest.

► Exhale to raise and straighten both legs in front of you.

► Inhale to bend the legs, returning the feet to the floor.

► Repeat eight times keeping the spine long.

ADDUCTOR ACTIVATION PRESSES

Alongside working with the roll of the inner thighs, it is possible to use this simple adductor isometric exercise to build strength and awareness.

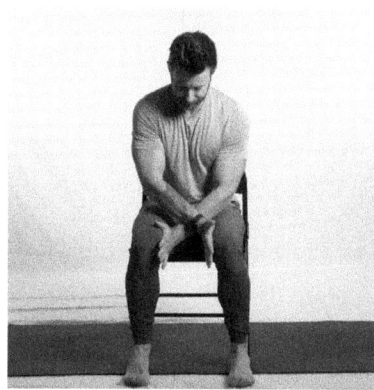

► Cross the arms at the wrists and set each palm on the opposite inner thigh, near the knee.

► Inhale to lengthen your spine and sit tall through the pelvis.

► Exhale to press the hands into the thighs as if to open them and resist by squeezing the thighs against the hands.

► Inhale to relax the pressure.

► Repeat this squeeze and release six times.

ABDUCTOR ACTIVATION PRESSES

Much like the adductor press above, learning how to switch on some of the muscles for abduction is important for the strength of the hips and the knees.

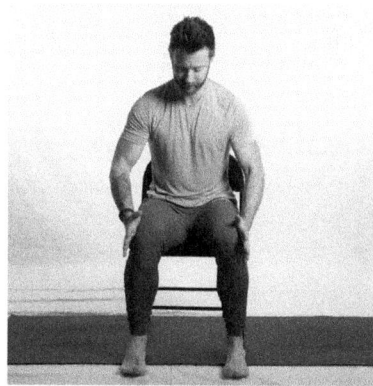

► Place the palms of the hands outside of the knees.

► Inhale to lengthen the spine and sit tall through the pelvis.

► Exhale to press the thighs outwards against the hands and resist with the hands. Keep the feet still.

► Inhale to relax the pressure.

► Repeat this six times.

SHOULDER RELIEVER

This pose combines both the abduction in the thighs with a shoulder opener. The pressing action in the legs causes an indirect spread on the upper back, which can be hard to achieve fully in poses like eagle.

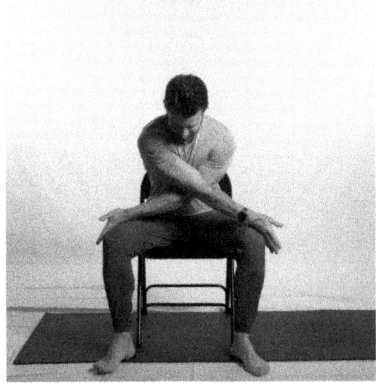

▶ Start with the feet slightly wider apart than hip distance.

▶ Place the back of each hand on the opposite knee.

▶ Inhale to lengthen the spine forwards.

▶ Exhale to press outwards with the thighs, allowing the shoulders to relax. Some tension is required in the hands and wrists to maintain the connection point.

▶ Hold for eight breaths. Take deep breaths that move the upper back.

UNLOCKING THE SHOULDERS – SINGLE ARM

This method is used to teach how to wrap the shoulder blades forwards as in the basic moves. This gets the shoulder blades moving on the back and allows isometric engagement of the chest and underarm muscles.

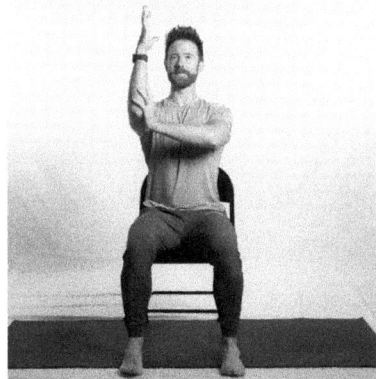

▶ Bring your arms up to shoulder height in front of you and bend the right arm 90 degrees so that your forearm is perpendicular to the floor. Bend the left arm and place the left palm on the inside of the right elbow.

▶ Inhale to telescope the ribs up.

▶ Exhale to draw the right shoulder back and down.

► Inhale to reach the elbow forwards, spreading the right shoulder blade wide.

► Exhale to press the hand into the elbow and elbow into the hand flexing your chest muscles. Hold for six breaths and repeat on the other side.

UNLOCKING THE SHOULDERS – BOTH ARMS

Working both arms allows you to get a sense of how to protract the upper back and create a sense of symmetry across the shoulder girdle.

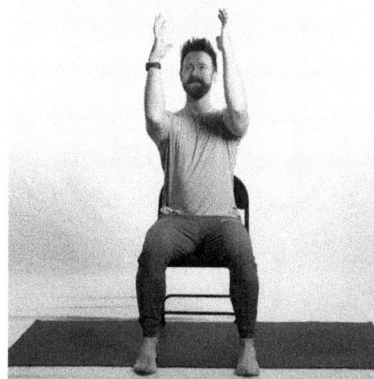

► Bring both arms up to shoulder height, and bend the elbows 90 degrees with the upper arms parallel to the floor and the forearms perpendicular to the floor.

► Inhale to telescope the ribs up.

► Exhale to draw the shoulders back and down.

► Inhale to reach the elbows forwards, spreading the shoulder blades wide.

► Exhale to squeeze the elbows in flexing your chest muscles. Hold for six breaths.

BIRD WING

When the posture of the upper back rounds forwards, our internal rotators (pectoralis minor) roll the shoulder heads forwards, and the ability to sense and use our external rotators becomes more of a challenge. Building awareness here is a great step towards having a healthy shoulder girdle and beginning the work of stabilising the shoulders. Using a resistance band between the hands can help build strength and tone here.

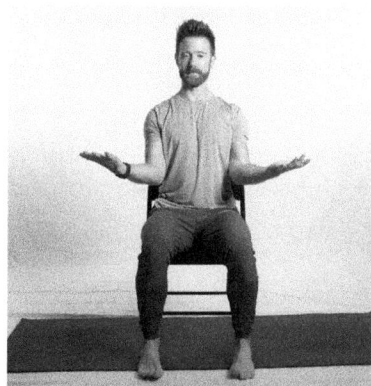

- Bend the elbows to 90 degrees, reach the forearms forward so they are parallel to the floor and turn the palms to face up.

- Nestle the elbows tightly against the rib cage.

- Inhale with the forearms parallel to the floor in front of you.

- Exhale to squeeze the elbows against the ribs and rotate the arms outwards so the palms move away from each other.

- Inhale to bring the arms back to parallel and repeat seven more times.

WEIGHTED SHRUGS

Seated shoulder shrugs are a great introduction to the squeeze and spread of the shoulder blades. As familiarity is found (in shoulder shrugs), adding a little more weight can help with the mobility of the upper back. This can either be done in plank as pictured or with the feet under the hips and hands under the shoulders for less resistance.

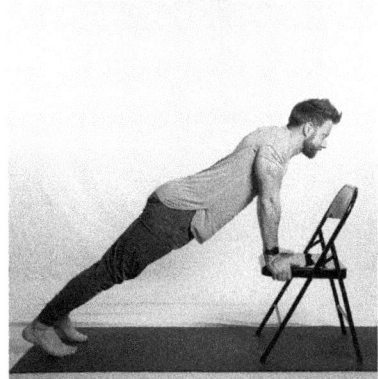

- With the hands on the seat of the chair, step back until the feet are either stacked underneath the hips or in a plank position. The hands should stay under the shoulders.

- Inhale to look forwards and lengthen the spine forwards.

- Exhale to draw the shoulder blades back as if they could touch, without moving the spine or ribcage.

- Inhale to push into the hands to spread the shoulder blades to their maximum without dropping the head.

- Repeat ten times.

CHAPTER FOUR

CORE WORK

There is a lot of thought about the core in the yoga and fitness world. Movement systems encourage a held core, engaged throughout almost every exercise, but this limits the reflective and instinctive functions of the core. In a lot of yoga practices, an idea of 'bandha' gets translated into 'locking', and rigidity seems to be what is left. Our society has placed particular emphasis on the appearance of the abdomen and midriff, and it has spilled into the visual representations we see in the online yoga world.

As we navigate this section, I want you to know that we are looking to maintain a relaxed core during our practice except when we are doing core work and are deliberately activating certain parts of the abdominal structures. We aren't looking to create more hardness and tension but, rather, a reflexive and responsive core so that when we lift the ribs and lengthen the spine, the core kicks in to support the action. Ideally, the core should be relaxed enough for abdominal breathing and long enough to be able to engage (thus my fascination with making sure back bending is part of your practice).

While your core will be used in many and all movements in a yoga practice, building a healthy relationship with this area is important, especially in determining what actions help to switch on the various muscular components of the core. The key is learning where they are, how to use them and how they can support your body in both your practice and your daily life.

The following pose suggestions may need less of a repetition count initially as you build familiarity with them. Over time, you may end up working higher counts of repetition and depth. With this enhanced mental representation, all poses hereafter will feel enhanced with greater awareness and understanding. This will be particularly evident when we get to twisting poses and side bends.

ABS WITH A ROLL

This is a great way to engage the core, mobilise the lower back and build strength and support at the inner thighs. If you don't have a foam roll, a block can be used here instead, but a rolled-up mat is a little softer. It will take a few rounds to get a feel for the order of events, but you could factor these into every practice from here on out. This has the added bonus of engaging a vital group of muscles, the adductors!

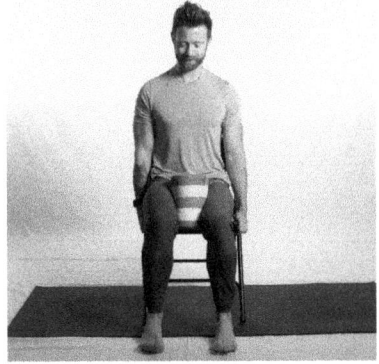

▶ Sitting straight, move the lower back away from the backrest of the chair. Inhale to lengthen the spine upwards.

▶ Exhale to tuck the pelvis down (ideally with little lower back movement) and squeeze the rolled-up mat. Repeat eight to ten times.

ALTERNATING LEG LIFTS

The hip flexors (the muscles that assist with lifting the legs) and the core are deeply linked. This exercise allows you to use manual resistance with your hand to create some engagement that will support the actions of the hips and support the lower back. This can be performed in a parallel position or in a wider stance while seated.

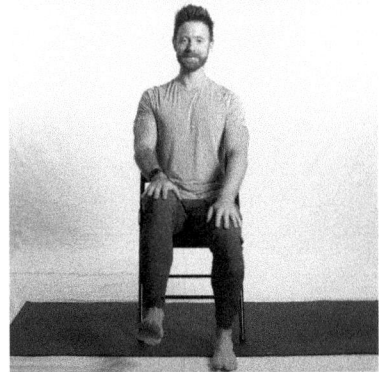

▶ Inhale to lengthen the spine upwards.

▶ Exhale to lift one leg, with the knee bent, press the hand on the same side into the thigh to create resistance and pull the abdomen inwards.

▶ Inhale to set the foot down, lengthening the spine, and repeat on the other side. Repeat fully four more times.

ALTERNATING LEG LIFTS WITH ARM AND LEG EXTENSION

Once you feel comfortable with the previous exercise, you can add in this contralateral exercise, which increases the demand on the core for stability. To challenge yourself further, sit away from the backrest of the chair.

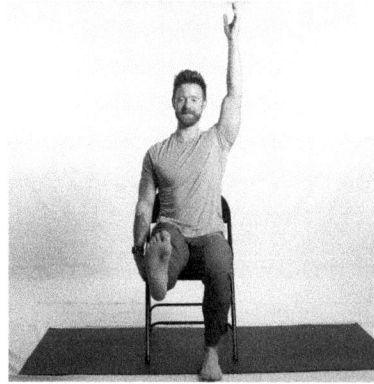

▶ Inhale to lengthen your spine upwards.

▶ Exhale to lift one foot, extending the leg forwards and straight, and raising the opposite arm straight up while pulling the abdomen inwards.

▶ Inhale to release the arm and leg down and repeat on the other side. Repeat four times.

OBLIQUE CRUNCH

I've called this a crunch but let's not crunch anything! Especially if you are low-back sensitive, a little goes a long way for this one. Focus on the sensation of the ribs moving towards the pelvis rather than simply leaning to the side. It should feel very active and deliberate. The hands can either be behind the head or crossed on the chest.

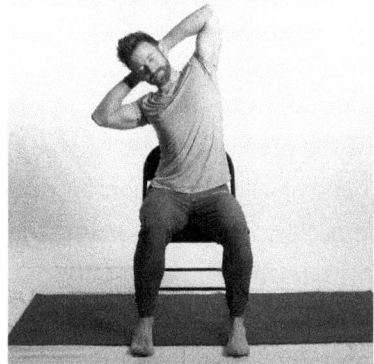

▶ Inhale to lengthen the spine upwards.

▶ Exhale to side bend to the right, bringing the ribs slightly closer to the pelvis.

▶ Inhale to lift back up and repeat on the other side.

▶ Repeat eight times per side.

OBLIQUE CRUNCH IN HORSE

This is identical to the previous oblique movement except for the variation in leg position. In a wide-leg stance, the relationship to the hip flexors can change, and if you are back sensitive, you gain the ability to stabilise the action by pushing down actively into the feet. The hands can either be behind the head or crossed on the chest.

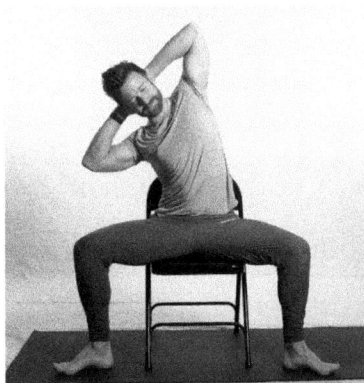

▶ Start with the legs wide apart. Inhale to lengthen the spine upwards.

▶ Exhale to side bend to the right, bringing the ribs slightly closer to the pelvis.

▶ Inhale to lift back up and repeat on the other side.

▶ Repeat eight times per side.

NAVASANA PREP

For this pose, you will need to sit on the chair side on, as the backrest blocks the movement of the pose. This pose will help you to start to build up your hip flexors and rectus abdominus muscles. Start by lessening the weight in the feet, raising the heels with the toes touching the ground and leaning back.

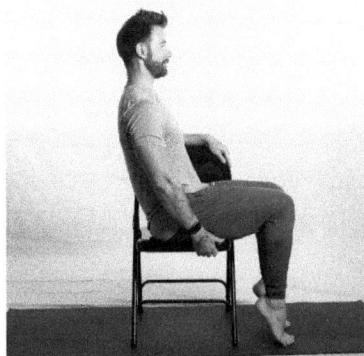

▶ Inhale to lift up out of the lower back.

▶ Exhale to pull the abdominal muscles in without rounding the back.

▶ Use the hands to support, especially if the lower back is uncomfortable.

▶ Aim to hold for eight breaths.

NAVASANA

Take care with the balance in this pose. Once strength is developed in the preparatory stage, you can build towards lifting the shin bones parallel to the floor.

Work with the feet and knees hip distance apart to give the hip flexors space.

It can take some time in the preparatory stage to build the strength and familiarity needed to lift the legs up without compromising the lower back.

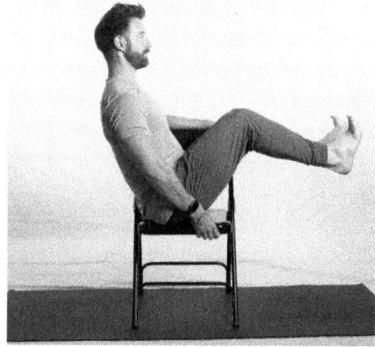

▶ Start in the preparatory stage and then lift the lower legs up.

▶ Inhale to lift up out of the lower back.

▶ Exhale to pull the abdominal muscles in without rounding the back.

▶ Use the hands to support, especially if the lower back is uncomfortable.

▶ Aim to hold for eight breaths.

CHAPTER FIVE

FORWARD BENDS

I often think of posture and movement as a diet, and I like to look at where food groups are missing and what needs scaling back. When seated, the body is already in a kind of forward bend with the hips flexed, with a tendency towards anterior head carriage – the head falling forwards of the shoulders – accompanied by a rounding of the upper back. So, if the diet is already rich in forward-bend nutrients, we need to mix things up a little bit, which is why there are so many more practices in Chapter Three on warming up and Chapter Nine on dynamic movement than in this chapter. Here, I hope to present various ways of moving the spine using a long spine – opening up the body in a way that facilitates movement in the lumbar and thoracic spine and alleviates tension in the back muscles. But forward bending should always be mixed in with back bends and twists, just to make sure that the diet doesn't lean towards one single element. That would be like trying to thrive on just potatoes every day!

Here you will find poses referring to both spinal flexion and hamstring work. I distinguish between the two, as it is very possible to forward bend and not really feel a stretch in the hamstrings and equally possible to work the hamstrings and not flex the spine. For me, given my experience with chronic lower-back disc problems, navigating into forward bends to feel the hamstrings more than the lower back is always my aim, but this requires the recruitment of the muscles of the lower back and mid/upper back (your erectors).

Visualising the back of the body – from the calves, the backs of the knees, hamstrings, pelvis, lower back and the spinal muscles up to the neck – our warm-up can help to move and lubricate for easier forward bending. Tension in any of these areas can make for difficulty in all forward-bending poses. So, here follows various poses and variations to help you navigate different parts of the back of the body.

When working in these poses, deep abdominal breathing is very useful to stop the abdomen from being rigid. The pressure changes that deep diaphragmatic breathing causes are profound and allow sensation and expansion in the lower back and at either side of the spine.

A blend of symmetrical to one-sided poses also helps us to learn if one side has developed different patterns from the other so we gain awareness in how to navigate many other poses. With the glutes and hamstrings contributing so much to lower back pain and hip pain, working one side at a time can also help reduce the pressure if a forward bend over both sides is too strenuous.

Given the direction of travel, learning to use your abdominals to deepen the contraction forwards and to navigate abdominal compression (the abdomen against the thighs, for example), core work is advised before delving into forward bends. Spinal movements like cat arches are also a great way to build up towards comfort and ease in forward bends.

In this section, given how muscles control the relationship of the spine to the pelvis and to gravity, we will work specific muscles. The muscles relating to posture will be classed as primary structural muscles, and muscles that move the limbs and have less of a direct effect on posture will be classed as secondary muscles. This classification usually helps in learning the where and why of the poses.

When looking at forward bending, we are speaking to the erector spinae group (iliocostalis, longissimus and spinalis) of the back and the rhomboids (rhomboid major and rhomboid minor). If these are tight, the conversation has to start at the hamstrings (semimembranosus, bicep femoris and semitendinosus). Staying with the back line of the body, we also have the gluteus maximus and the piriformis determining the neutral tilt of the pelvis and the ability to rotate the thighs. So we see a blend of primary structural muscles and secondary ones in play with the back body.

FORWARD BEND WITH A BLANKET

The folded blanket on the lap allows for a gentle pressure into the abdomen. The aim is to be fairly relaxed in this forward bend, unlike some of the other more active versions in this chapter. By using deep breaths directed towards the abdomen, the pressure change in the abdominal cavity moves the lower back, stimulates the pelvic floor and stretches the tissues of the mid and upper back. Deep breathing with abdominal pressure can even stetch the rhomboids.

▶ Start with the feet hip distance apart. Fold the blanket and place it on both thighs. Inhale to lengthen the spine.

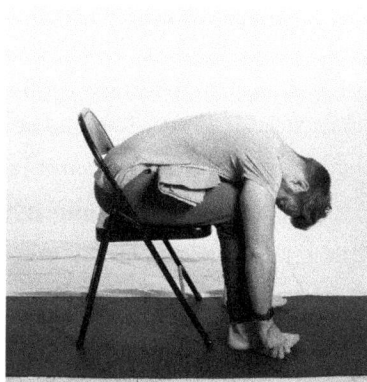

▶ Exhale to fold from the hips over the thighs and relax the arms down, with the neck relaxed.

▶ For ease of access, if you are able to sit forwards in the chair, there will be more available space to fold.

▶ Hold for eight breath cycles and take your time exiting the pose.

FORWARD BEND WITH BLOCKS

This pose can be done in a parallel foot position or with the feet wider apart to accommodate the need for more space or if the legs are uncomfortable folding when seated in the chair (sometimes the firmness can block the movement of the legs). Position two blocks outside of the feet or to the inside if in a wider stance.

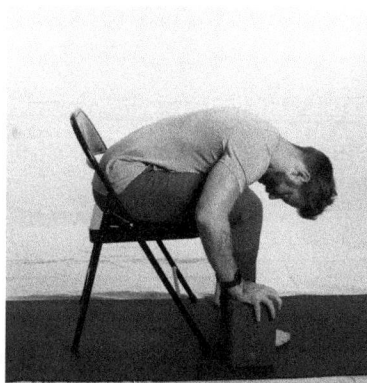

▶ Inhale to lift the chest forwards and up.

▶ Exhale to fold forwards until the hands are on the blocks. Feel free to move the blocks lower (so that the long side is touching the floor).

▶ Inhale and lengthen the low front ribs forwards, away from your pelvis.

▶ Exhale to relax your neck and stick your butt out.

▶ Stay for eight breaths and slowly come up to seated.

FORWARD BEND WITH A BOLSTER

This is a very passive forward bend, where instead of actively trying to lengthen the ribs forwards or activate the lower back, the aim is to rest and relax some of the body's heavy lifting muscles. If you don't have a bolster, a second chair with a pillow on it would be soft enough to work. This can be done in a wide or narrow stance (as pictured).

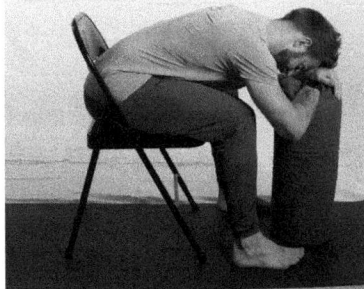

► Hinge forwards from the hips and relax the arms onto a bolster placed upright in front of the body. If possible, allow the head to rest on the hands to take the pressure off your spinal muscles.

► Rest here for ten breaths.

HALFWAY LIFT ON BLOCKS

From a forward bend on blocks, we can add in this halfway lift. The purpose here is to engage the back of the body to create a long and flatter spine rather than the deep fold we have come from to get a good balance of postural movement. This is about engaging the erectors; even the neck is active in this pose. This can be performed narrow as pictured or in a wide stance.

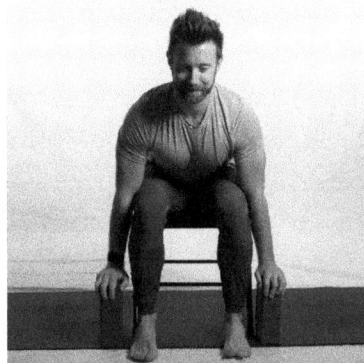

► In the seated fold with the hands on blocks next to the feet, inhale to scoop the chest forwards, lengthening the spine forwards. Press down into active feet and stick your butt out as much as you can.

► Hold for eight breaths or alternate between the fold and the halfway lift for eight repetitions.

FORWARD BEND WITH NECK TRACTION

Spinal decompression is one of the main reasons we employ the 'telescope the ribs'/'tuck the tailbone' basic moves. In this forward bend, the chair anchors the pelvis and allows the head and neck to lengthen towards the floor, creating a spinal traction.

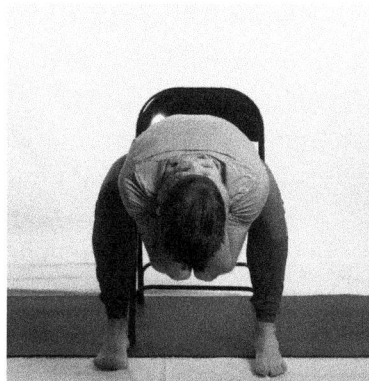

▶ Start in a wider than hip distance stance. Clasp the hands at the back of the neck and try to tap the elbows together under the chin.

▶ Exhale to fold forwards from the hips and endeavour to reach the elbows downwards, with the neck relaxed (even though it is held).

▶ Hold for ten breaths.

SINGLE LEG HOLD WITH A STRAP (STAGE 1)

The next four poses use a strap to help isolate each leg. For balance, each one will affect the hamstrings on both the inner and outer aspects of the thighs, including the inner thighs, which can feel like tight hamstrings when they are tight. It is important that the upper body is as relaxed as possible when using the strap.

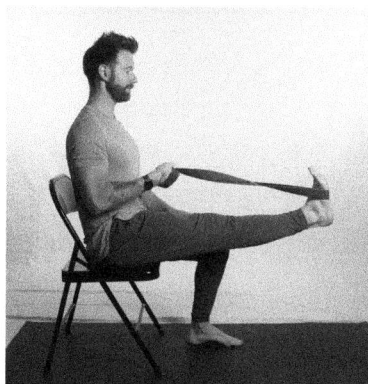

▶ In a seated position, loop the strap under one foot around the arch.

▶ Either sitting straight up or against the frame of the chair, lift this leg until it is straight.

▶ Inhale to telescope the spine up.

▶ Exhale to stick your butt out and flex the foot (toes pull towards you).

▶ Hold for eight breaths.

THIGH ADDUCTION (STAGE 2)

Not only does this help stretch the outermost hamstring, but it also creates a stretch on the gluteus medius and a little on the piriformis, relieving pressure on the hip. This can sometimes feel a bit nervy, but persevere!

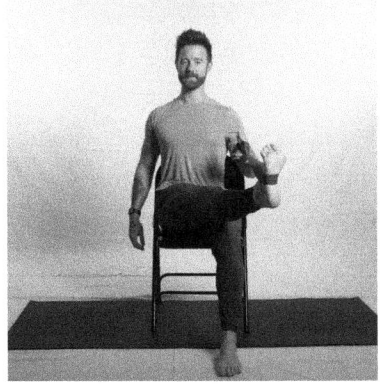

▶ In a seated position, loop the strap under one foot around the arch.

▶ Either sitting straight up or against the frame of the chair, lift this leg until it is straight.

▶ Inhale to telescope the spine up.

▶ Exhale to pull the leg towards the other leg (it may not move very much), keeping the pelvis still.

▶ Hold for eight breaths.

THIGH ABDUCTION (STAGE 3)

Sharing a neighbouring insertion point with the hamstrings, the inner thigh muscles (gracilis) and rotators (sartorius) when tight can feel like tight hamstrings, so working them together when targeting the hamstrings is a good plan.

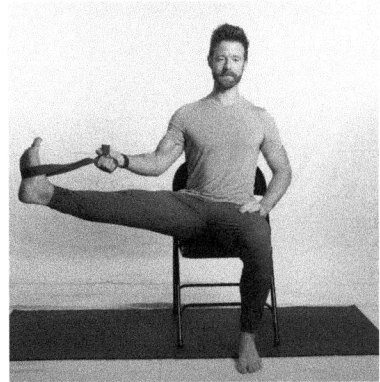

▶ In a seated position, loop the strap under one foot around the arch.

▶ Either sitting straight up or against the frame of the chair, lift this leg until it is straight.

▶ Inhale to telescope the spine up.

▶ Exhale to pull the leg outwards to the side, away from the body, keeping the pelvis still.

▶ Hold for eight breaths.

TWISTING TRIANGLE (STAGE 4)

Adding extra tension and movement forces to a pose can deepen the sensation. Adding a twist into our stage 1 pose allows for an increased awareness of the pelvis position and an increase in tension down the outside of the thigh to stretch the iliotibial (IT) band, vastus lateralis and tensor fasciae latae (TFL), helping to take pressure off the knee and hip of that side.

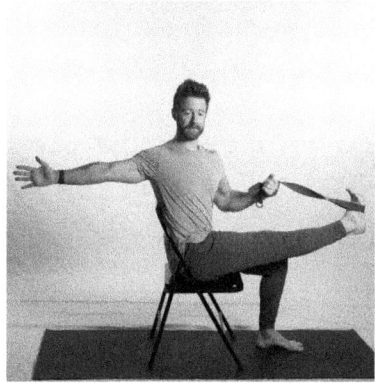

▶ In a seated position, loop the strap under one foot around the arch and hold the strap with the opposite hand.

▶ Either sitting straight up or against the frame of the chair, lift this leg until it is straight.

▶ Inhale to telescope the spine up.

▶ Exhale to twist towards the lifted leg, reach the arm back, and take care not to pull the lifted leg across the opposite thigh.

▶ Hold for eight breaths.

STANDING FORWARD BEND

This is quite a passive forward bend with bent legs to help stretch the hamstrings and create an inversion quality. Using the chair means you can rest the arms or hands at various height levels. With a wider stance, this can also be used for a standing straddle forward bend.

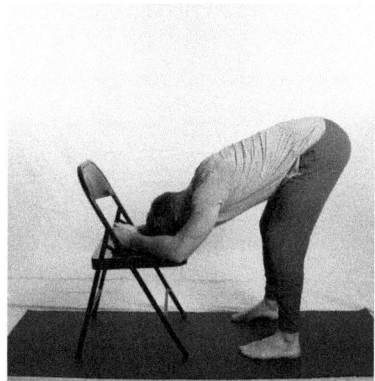

▶ Facing the chair, with the feet hip distance apart or slightly wider, bend the knees.

▶ Inhale to lengthen the ribs up.

▶ Exhale to hinge from the hips, sticking your butt out to initiate the movement, and rest the hands on the chair. Keep the neck relaxed.

▶ Stay here for eight breaths.

ACTIVE STANDING FORWARD BEND

Unlike the previous pose, this pose is about active recruitment of the back muscles, which creates a long and strong spine. Especially if you find that your lower back gets irritated by forward bends, this is a great way to stretch the hamstrings without rounding the spine. If the hands go too low, the lower back will probably take the stretch rather than the hamstrings.

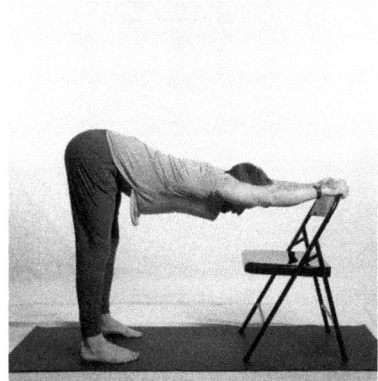

▶ Facing the chair, with the feet hip distance apart or slightly wider, bend the knees.

▶ Inhale to lengthen the ribs up.

▶ Exhale to hinge from the hips, sticking the butt out to initiate the movement, and rest the hands on the high backrest.

▶ Inhale to telescope the ribs towards the chair and stick your butt out.

▶ Exhale, and gradually straighten the legs without rounding the back.

▶ Stay here for eight breaths.

SINGLE LEG FORWARD BEND

▶ Using the support of the chair, we can isolate one leg at a time, reducing the overall
pressure on the back. This is also a great
way to experiment with flexed foot positions to stretch into the calf and back of the
knee, which share an intimate relationship
with the hamstrings.

▶ Sitting on the edge of the chair, straighten
the right leg forwards on the ground and flex
the foot. Anchor the left foot to the floor for
balance. Place one or two blocks under the hands to help with leaning forwards.

▶ Inhale to lengthen the chest towards the right foot.

▶ Exhale to stick your butt out, drawing the toes towards the knee, with the toes
tracking straight up.

▶ Hold for eight breaths and repeat on the other side.

▶ For variation, explore doing a round with the front foot turned out to stretch
the outermost hamstring and one round with the foot turned in to stretch the
two innermost hamstrings.

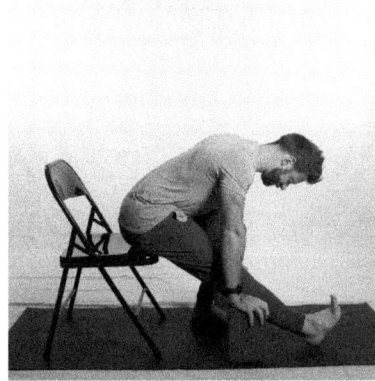

PYRAMID

Much like the seated forward fold, this allows
us to stretch the back of one leg while maintaining a long spine. In classes, this is frequently
instructed with the feet lined up with each
other. To effectively articulate the pelvis and
lower back, the feet need to be hip width apart.

▶ Start facing the chair, with the feet hip distance apart. Fold forwards to hold the top
frame of the chair. Step one leg back about
two to three feet.

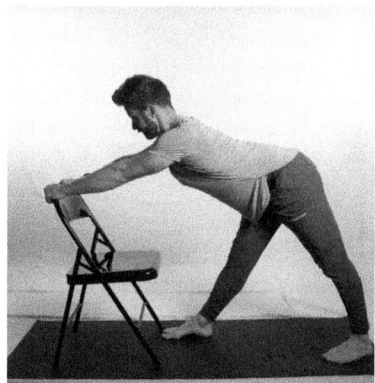

▶ To keep the back long, the front leg may need to bend considerably.

▶ Inhale to lengthen the chest towards the chair, pressing the back of the skull upwards.

▶ Exhale to stick your butt out and actively press into the front foot.

▶ Hold for eight breaths and repeat on the other side.

▶ For variation, explore doing a round with the front foot turned out to stretch the outermost hamstring and one round with the foot turned in to stretch the two innermost hamstrings.

CHAPTER SIX

BACK BENDS

Back bends have a very different feel to the introverted and soothing qualities of forward bends. These poses invigorate and open the chest, building endurance in the back muscles that support your posture. Where forward bends can exacerbate the forward slump of the head and shoulders, back bending allows for both the stretching of the muscles that pull the shoulders forwards and the strengthening of muscles that challenge the effects of prolonged sitting. In strengthening the upper back, stretching the quads and hip flexors, we find the antidote for our natural postural tendency of folding forwards.

Strengthening the back, moving the upper spine and navigating chest opening poses means the rib cage can become more flexible. With increased rib cage flexibility, there will also be respiratory benefits, allowing for a more comfortable deep breath.

Creating movement in the shoulders and arms, openness in the chest muscles, mobility of the spine and relief of the hip flexors (the front of the hips) contributes to the back-bending poses you will meet in this chapter. When working the shoulder, the relationship with the neck is also important, with many muscles sharing connections with the head, neck and shoulder. In my own practice, I like to start with smaller back bends and build up as the body warms up. Significant warm-up is required for back bends, with a focus on shoulders, spinal movement and even hip warm-up.

Normally, in a yoga class, there is the pattern of doing a counter pose in the opposite direction; for example, after a forward bend, do a back bend – and the reverse. When we look at spinal movement, though, I find it best to work a theme, gradually building up back bends and then taking time to bring the spine back towards a neutral position. Back tractions, side bends, twists and then hip opening all help bring the spinal position back to a comfortable equilibrium. When we get to Chapter Fourteen, you will see how a sequence can build safely into bigger back bends, with a warm-down factored in too.

Much like forward bending, the direction of movement demands that some postural muscles engage and others lengthen. Given that a lot of practices are heavily weighted towards forward bending, and that it is the natural default position of sitting, back bends are worth their weight in gold.

Moving into external shoulder rotation positions requires some awareness and strength in the muscles that rotate the arm and change the position of the shoulder blade (supraspinatus, infraspinatus, teres minor and teres major), combined with openness in pectoralis minor. A tight pectoralis minor contributes to the forward rolling of the humerus and forward carriage of the head.

This section will also begin the work of freeing up the neck, especially the scalenes (anterior, middle and posterior). These contribute to pressure in the brachial plexus (which enervates the arms) and phrenic nerve (which enervates the diaphragm), making them important muscles to lengthen and strengthen.

Our other primary structural muscle that can be lengthened in back bends is the psoas major, sometimes called *the* structural muscle, with its capacity to compress more nerves than most other muscles. When tight, it compresses the lower back, rounds the upper body and can even push the abdominal organs forwards. It is also a primary muscle in determining whether the pelvis is in a posterior or anterior tilt, much like the hamstrings and erectors.

CHEST OPENING POSE

Chest opening pose is a great passive pose to explore rib cage flexibility and the mobility required for overhead reaching that we will use in some of the other back bends. If you don't have a bolster, a second chair or windowsill could work well. When done with the elbows on the bolster, you can recreate the sensations of dolphin, which you will meet later in this chapter.

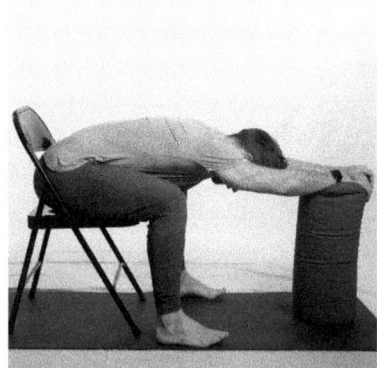

- In a wide stance, place the bolster a few feet away from the chair; it will seem quite far away, but the reach is the combined length of your arms and torso.

- Exhale to lean forwards, placing the hands or forearms on the bolster.

- Inhale to shrug the shoulder blades up towards your ears.

- Exhale to hang the chest downwards with the neck relaxed.

- Hold for ten breaths.

SINGLE ARM CHEST OPENING

Much like the previous pose, this creates a focus on one side of the body. Exploring the differences between the sides can be very important when developing a regular practice. Sometimes the rib cage does all the work here. Aim for the collarbones to remain level and parallel to the floor.

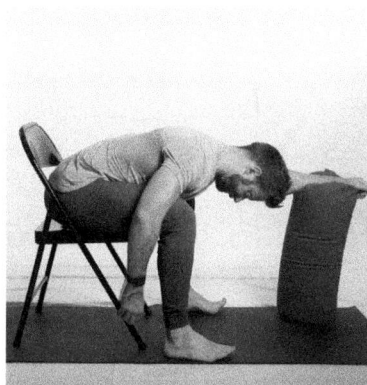

- In a wide stance, place the bolster a few feet away from the chair.

- Exhale to lean forwards, placing one hand or forearm on the bolster. Let the other arm hang down by the side of the leg.

- Inhale to shrug the shoulder blade on the supported side up towards your ears.

- Exhale to hang the chest downwards with the neck relaxed.

- Hold for ten breaths and repeat on the other side.

NECK RELEASE

This and the next pose help to open and stretch the chest muscles, the front of the shoulder and the neck to assist later with back bends. When pectoralis minor is tight, it can pull the shoulders forwards. When stretched, it can begin to relieve the chronic tension in these muscles. Angling the chin up can also create stretch in the scalenes but may be accompanied by tingling in the hand.

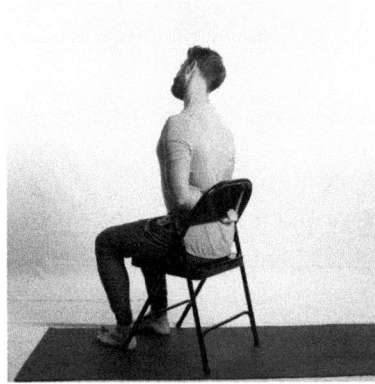

- ▶ Leave a little space between your back and the chair.

- ▶ Bring the right arm behind your back to hold the frame of the chair or your waistband.

- ▶ Exhale to draw the right shoulder blade back slightly and relax the neck to the left.

- ▶ Hold for eight breaths.

- ▶ Repeat with the left arm behind the back.

NECK RELEASE (ARM HOLD)

This neck release encourages a little more flexibility in the shoulders but creates a slightly different tension across the chest muscles and collarbones.

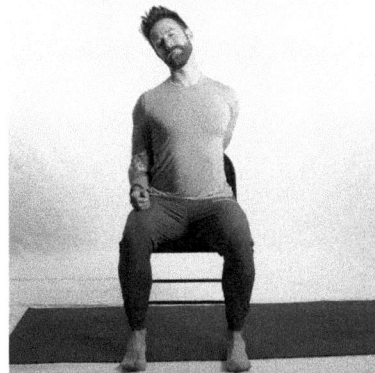

- ▶ Leave a little space between your back and the chair.

- ▶ Bring the left arm behind your back to hold

the crook of the right elbow (if you can't reach, hold the frame of the chair or waistband).

▶ Exhale to draw the left shoulder blade back slightly and relax the neck to the right.

▶ Hold for eight breaths.

▶ Repeat with the right arm behind the back.

DOLPHIN

This is a fantastic chest opening pose, giving an opportunity to lower the mid back down towards the ground, creating a back bend. In addition, the overhead reach with bent arms allows both the triceps and latissimus dorsi muscles to be stretched. When at the depth of the pose, even a deep breath will be challenging against the stretching chest area.

The pose can be replicated in a similar manner to chest opening pose by placing the elbows onto the bolster.

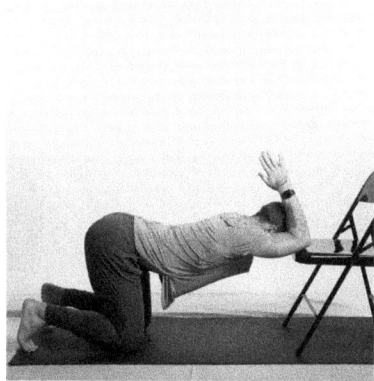

▶ Use the chair to transition in a comfortable kneeling position on the floor, facing the chair, with the knees torso distance away from the chair. Place the elbows on the chair with the forearms pointing straight up and palms together overhead. Stack the hips above the knees; this may require a bit of a shuffle.

▶ Exhale to lower the chest towards the ground and then bend the elbows, with the neck relaxed between the arms.

▶ Hold for eight breaths.

BRIDGE WITH A ROLL

While this pose was also in the warm-up section, this is also a great back bending pose and one I recommend doing daily! It creates a strong foundation in the legs and inner thighs, and a bit of space in the front of the hips, and then adds in a chest opener. If you used the pose in the warm-up, try adding it in a little later on to see what has changed as you have been practising.

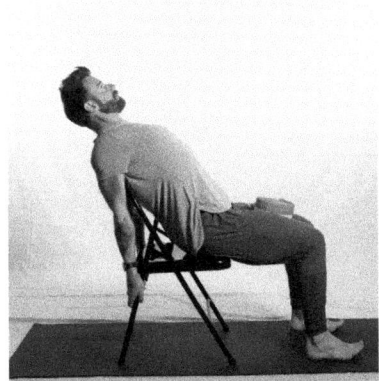

▶ Slide forwards on the chair so you can lean back a little. Place a roll between the thighs. Press into active feet until you feel your hamstrings kick in, but take care not to push backwards.

▶ Inhale to lengthen the ribs away from the pelvis.

▶ Exhale to squeeze the roll, taking the arms down by your side to hold the rear legs of the chair.

▶ Hold for ten breaths.

CHAIR POSE

Developing strength in the erectors is an important part of postural development, and chair pose (utkatasana) offers a great challenge for that. By actively sticking the butt out, the main heavy lifters of the back, from the lower back to the skull, will kick in. There is also the option to test the balance by leaning forwards to see if the butt can lift from the chair (but this is not necessary).

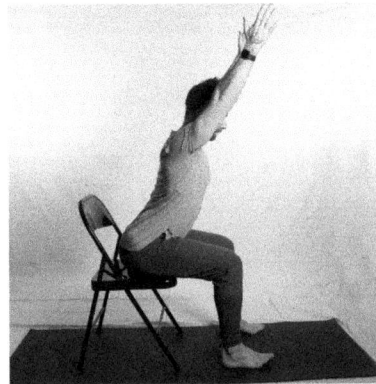

- ▶ Create some space between the rear of the chair and your pelvis/spine and set the feet hip distance apart.

- ▶ Inhale to reach the arms forwards and up, shoulder width apart.

- ▶ Exhale to stick your butt out and press the skull backwards without lifting the chin.

- ▶ Hold for eight breaths.

LUNGE

Like bridge, this is a staple pose on the path towards alignment of the bones. By allowing the spine to be neutral and working that 'tuck tailbone down' action, it is possible to stretch the quads and hip flexors, areas that are noto- riously tight. Side-facing presents a balance issue, so make sure that you feel secure and hold on to the chair back.

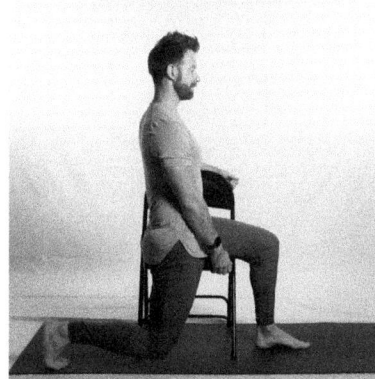

- ▶ Pivot in the chair to face the left side. Move the left leg until the knee is also facing left.

- ▶ Allow the right leg to internally rotate until the knee is under the hip; it does not need to touch the floor.

- ▶ Inhale to telescope the ribs up and press down into both feet.

- ▶ Exhale to tuck tailbone down.

- ▶ Hold for eight breaths and repeat on the other side.

CHEST OPENER

While this pose may look similar to bridge, it uses the backrest of the chair to assist the bend in the thoracic spine. It is recommended to place a blanket on top of a firm chair for comfort. Rather than allowing the head to fall backwards, maintain a bit of hold in the muscles in the front of the neck with a small chin tuck.

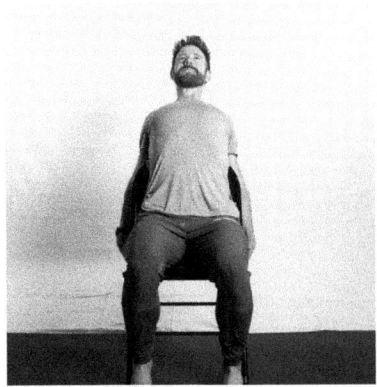

▶ Sit with your back against the frame of the chair and feet hip distance apart.

▶ Inhale to lift the arms up and lift the ribcage up.

▶ Exhale to circle the arms down to the sides of the chair, perhaps to hold the rear legs of the chair. Squeeze the shoulder blades together.

▶ Focus on deep breathing for eight breaths.

CACTUS ARMS BACK BEND

This back bend is a big rhomboid strengthener. Increasing the flexibility of the chest combined with strengthening the postural muscles of the upper back allows the shoulders the opportunity to rest in a more retracted state rather than falling forwards.

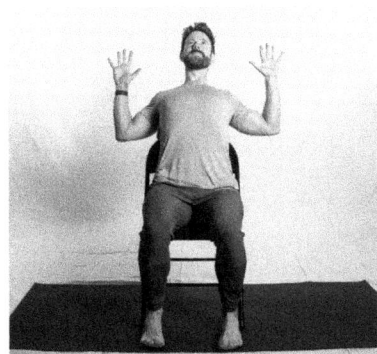

▶ In an upright seated position, place a blanket over the backrest of the chair.

▶ Inhale to telescope the ribs up, lifting the arms up.

▶ Exhale to bend the arms to the side, with the forearms pointing towards the ceiling, and squeeze the shoulder blades back with the palms facing forwards.

▶ Lean the upper back over the chair while maintaining a solid press down through the feet.

▶ Hold for eight breaths or move through the instructions with the breath repeatedly for eight rounds.

SINGLE ARM CHEST OPENER

This pose can be done away from a wall, but to really get the most out of this stretch, set your chair up near a wall, roughly a foot away. This is an important stretch for releasing chronic tension in pectoralis minor (one of the muscles responsible for the forward rolling of the shoulders). Don't be alarmed at tingling or numbness in the thumb, index and middle fingers, as this muscle sits over the nerve plexus.

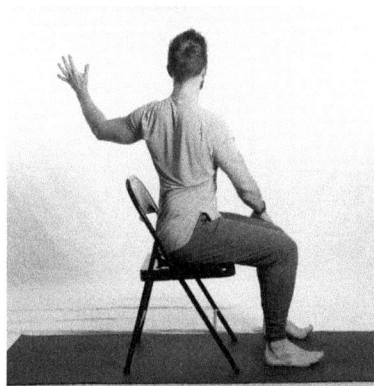

▶ Inhale to lift the ribcage up.

▶ Exhale to twist to the left, drawing the left arm back so the elbow is lower and further back than the shoulder (if at a wall, set the left hand flat to the wall), with the elbow bent.

▶ Inhale to telescope the ribs up.

▶ Exhale to slowly turn the chest back forwards.

▶ Hold for eight breaths and repeat on the other side.

BACK BEND WITH A STRAP

We met active archer in the warm-up; this pose allows for both arms to be involved while navigating the back bend. The chair in the photo has a backrest for the strap to thread through; if you don't have a chair like that, you can sit on the strap to keep it still. This pose allows for a very active press up, allowing the breastbone to shift forwards into the back bend.

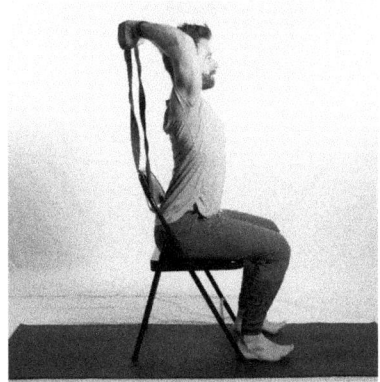

▶ Once you have the strap behind you (threaded through the back rest or you can sit on it), hold both ends of it roughly shoulder distance apart with the elbows bent.

▶ Inhale to push the fists up.

▶ Exhale to wrap the shoulder blades forwards a little and elevate the shoulders.

▶ Create tension in the strap and lean the chest forwards while remaining upright. If the arms straighten, slip the grip further down the strap.

▶ Hold for ten breaths.

STRAP CAMEL

This is a favourite of mine. If you are able to stand, this works really well with a gentle standing back bend. In most back bends, the neck has a bit of a hard time, as the muscles on the front of the neck may not be strong in supporting that direction, but when we create this support using a strap and a blanket, the head, neck and upper back can all move into an effortless back bend, so do tolerate the faff!

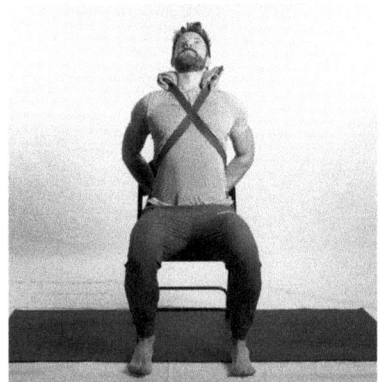

▶ Place the middle of the strap on the short

end of a blanket (or towel) and roll the blanket tightly around the strap until it is about a foot wide and a couple of inches thick. The strap should be held inside the rolled blanket. Place this support on the back of the neck, cross the strap at the breastbone, bring the ends around to the lower back and hold them with the hands at the lower back.

▶ Inhale to telescope the ribs up.

▶ Exhale to draw the elbows back, squeezing the shoulder blades towards each other.

▶ Inhale to lift the cross in the strap (breastbone).

▶ Exhale to relax the neck back against the roll support.

▶ Hold for ten breaths.

NECK TRACTION

Continuing our fun with straps, here is the neck traction back bend. If you have ever felt like you just needed your spine pulled long, this one is for you! Pulling upwards helps to switch on the shoulders while decompressing the back, something that can be a real challenge for folks new to back bends.

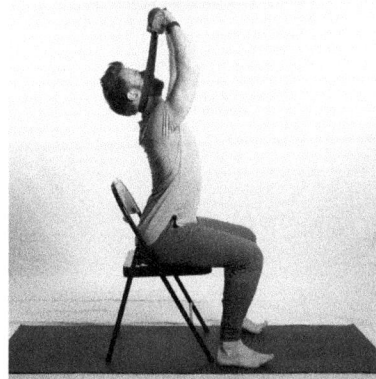

▶ Slip the strap behind the head at the occipital ridge and lean the head back.

▶ Hold the strap in each hand just far enough away that the arms are still bent.

▶ Inhale to telescope the ribs up.

▶ Exhale to wrap the shoulders forwards and pull upwards.

▶ Endeavour to relax the neck while pulling upwards into the back bend.

▶ Hold for eight breaths.

REVERSE TABLETOP

While this pose may take some time to build up to, I see it as a keystone pose for chest opening. With a combination of strength and front-body opening, this pose presents a wonderful counter pose to sitting. You will need a sturdy chair for this.

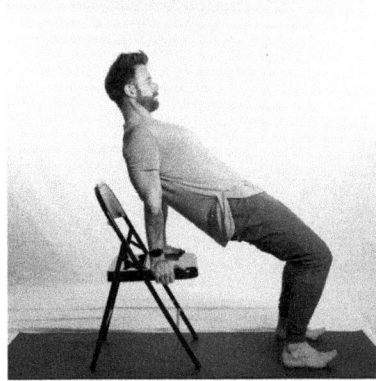

▶ While sitting on the front of the chair, take the hands behind you to hold the edges of the seat. Take the legs forwards until they are straight.

▶ Inhale to bend the legs, taking your weight off the chair and into the hands and legs.

▶ Exhale to press down into active feet and draw the shoulders back.

▶ Inhale to lift the ribcage up, lengthening the spine without allowing the head to fall backwards.

▶ Hold for ten breaths or lower and lift ten times.

DANCER

This pose is a balance; holding the chair can make a huge difference to the feel of the pose. By using an active push with the leg, and all of the shoulder work in this chapter, one can achieve a chest opener that feels like it integrates many of the movements we have focused on.

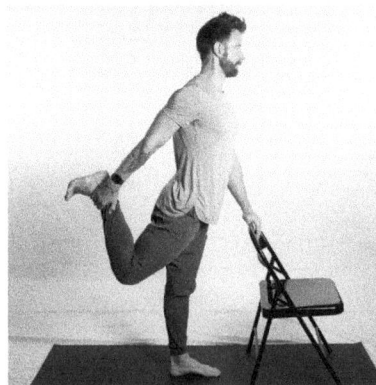

▶ Stand facing the back of the chair.

▶ Set the left hand onto the backrest of the chair.

▶ Exhale to lift the right knee forwards and up so you can grab the ankle and then draw the ankle behind the body. Alternatively, bend the right leg behind the body and reach back to the ankle with the right hand.

▶ Inhale to telescope the ribs up and square the pelvis and chest towards the chair.

▶ While holding the foot, exhale to push the leg back, drawing the right shoulder blade back as the chest squares forwards.

▶ Hold for eight breaths and repeat on the other side. If getting the ankle is a challenge, grab a strap to help.

UPWARD FACING DOG

One of the best things about this pose is that you can easily control the depth by how much you lower the hips. The lower the hips, the more flexibility will be demanded from the hips and lower back. This is such an important pose to relieve the pressure in the front of the hips (hip flexors).

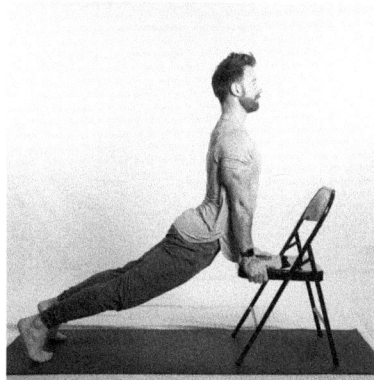

▶ Facing the chair, with the hands on its seat, step the feet back until there is a roughly 90 degrees hinge at the hips.

▶ Inhale to lean forwards, bringing the hips closer to the chair and moving onto the tiptoes.

▶ Exhale, draw the shoulders back and down away from the ears and tuck the tailbone down.

▶ Hold for eight breaths or shift back to the start position and into the pose with the breath eight times.

CHAPTER SEVEN

TWISTS

One of the main movements in any of the chair classes I run is rotation. These invigorating poses can feel very challenging at first, but they are also where I see people progress the fastest, as many of the jigsaw pieces come together. Almost all of these twists involve several major joints, from the hips to the shoulders, all of which are essential to many other yoga poses. For example, in a seated twist to the right, your right shoulder blade moves closer to the spine, contracting the muscles that attach the blade to the ribcage. The opposite shoulder blade moves further from the spine, creating a conversation with the shoulder girdle that helps realign the relationship between the limbs and the torso.

In the course of a sedentary life, our rotational axis becomes disrupted, and the spinal joint mobility and connective tissues can gradually shorten. Regular practice can help restore limitations in the core and the muscles of the spine, rib cage, upper back and hips.

The basic move of telescoping the ribs and lengthening the spine should be observed in any twist, regardless of the direction. As soon as the head falls forwards of the line of the shoulders (that anterior head carriage again), spinal rotation and deep beathing will be limited. Almost all of the twists in this section are active, inviting you to engage your muscles to support the pose rather than to sink in.

Discovering which spinal sections can move well is a big part of this, and in general, people who are hypermobile tend to move the pelvis and neck, with very little movement through the lower and middle back. The direction of rotational ability can also vary significantly with great variation between sides. In general, the neck is most capable of rotation, followed by the lower back and the mid back, due to the attached ribs and layers of muscle. To ensure the integrity of the sacroiliac joints and to maintain stability of the lower back, I recommend keeping the pelvis still and rotating on your axis from the lower spine up.

This section will look at twists on a vertical axis and a horizontal axis. This mix of both gives the muscles we use in twists an opportunity to resist the pull of gravity. This will challenge your back muscles, core and neck in a different way from seated, so it can be good to build up to these poses. Since the body is a weight-bearing entity with a gravitational field, proper balance between front and back, and left and right, is essential in keeping it pain free and functioning properly.

In my own practice, twists are where I have to be most cautious. As someone who is hypermobile, it is easy for me to twist from my lower back and move into the pelvis and sacroiliac joints, causing pain in these joints, which can show up a day or two later. As these joints experience forces or torsion, tension and rotation, this stiff joint provides shock absorption for the spine from the upper body to the lower body. Rather than going into extreme ranges, stabilising the pelvis (staying anchored through your sit bones), prioritising the mobility of the mid and upper spine and strengthening the core and legs can all help support these joints in the long term.

In this chapter, you will find a mix of poses that work dynamically and poses that are static and active. For balance, do a combination of both types of pose. You may find that some twists get easier to access when you do a dynamic warm-up drill before navigating them. For more complex poses that involve so many parts of the body, core work, as well as a thorough warm-up, should be part of your practice.

ACTIVE TWIST

Working with the hands behind the head and pressing the skull back into the hands (without lifting the chin) allows for the postural muscles of the neck and upper back to be switched on in anticipation of twisting. This can be really useful for finding that axis of rotation.

▶ Sit with some space between your back and the chair. Clasp the hands behind your head.

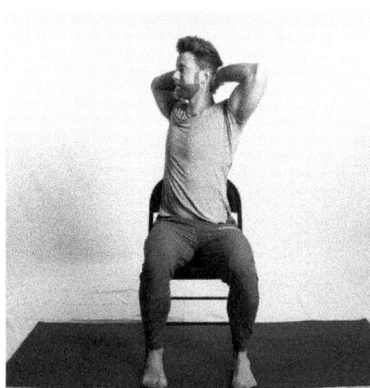

▶ Inhale to telescope the ribs up, pressing the head into the hands. Pull upwards on the skull.

▶ Exhale to twist to the right, keeping the pelvis still and anchored.

▶ Hold for eight breaths and repeat on the other side.

▶ This pose can also be done actively by moving into the twist on each exhale.

TWIST

When I lead classes, I usually sequence the previous twist straight into this one before changing sides. The proprioceptive awareness of having the hands behind the head helps to prevent the forwards drop of the head, keeping the spine aligned for this twist, which involves more of the upper back for leverage.

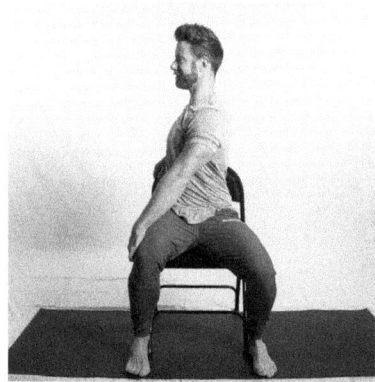

▶ In a seated position, leave some space between your back and the chair.

▶ Inhale to telescope the ribs and skull upwards.

▶ Exhale to twist to the right, taking the left hand to the right knee and the right hand behind onto the chair wherever is comfortable. Create a pulling action with both arms and a slight squeeze of the left shoulder blade towards the spine.

▶ Hold for eight breaths and repeat on the other side.

TWIST WITH HIPS

I usually work with this twist straight after the previous two. In it, we pivot 90 degrees to the side. This helps keep the pelvis (and therefore the lower back muscles) level while offering the opportunity to twist with both hands on the chair and working with one hip flexed and the other relaxed downwards to take pressure off the joint.

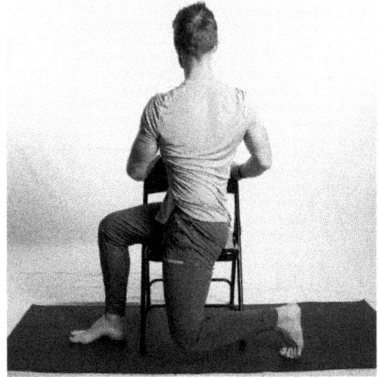

▶ In a seated position, leave some space between your back and the chair.

▶ Inhale to telescope the ribs and skull upwards.

▶ Exhale to twist to the left, pivoting to face the left side of the chair. Point the right knee downwards and hold the backrest of the chair. Create a pulling action with both arms and create a slight tuck down through the pelvis to stretch the front of the right hip.

▶ Hold for eight breaths and repeat on the other side.

ACTIVE TWIST WITH WIDE ARMS

Working with the arms open, rather than behind the head, challenges your active range of motion. The previous two poses have used the mechanical pulling actions of the arms to generate a passive twist; here, you can only go as far as you can go, and when you get there, breathing will be a challenge. The opportunity to strengthen the muscles of the upper back outweighs the challenge.

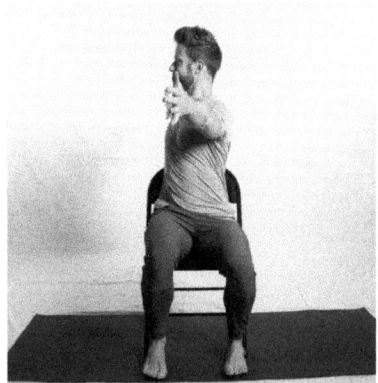

▶ Sit with some space between your back and

the chair. Open the arms out wide, with the shoulder blades relaxed into a neutral position.

▶ Inhale to telescope the ribs up.

▶ Exhale to twist to the right, keeping the pelvis still and anchored. The arms should stay in line with the collarbones.

▶ Hold for eight breaths and repeat on the other side.

▶ This pose can also be done actively by moving into the twist on each exhale.

CHAIR POSE TWIST 1

Much like utkatasana when we met it in Chapter Six on back bends, this is a great way to feel how the legs can support and create a foundation for rotation. The next four poses build on each other, offering more rotation and changes of leverage.

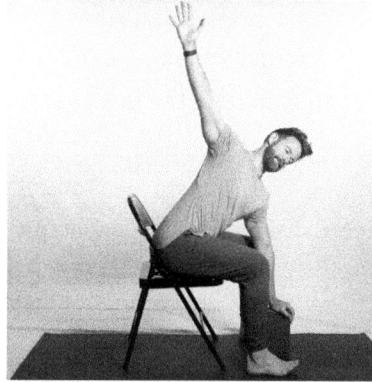

▶ In a parallel stance for the lower body, lean forwards so both hands are on a block placed between the feet.

▶ Inhale to telescope the spine forwards away from the hips.

▶ Exhale to twist to the right, lifting the right arm; aim to keep the pelvis as still as possible.

▶ Either hold for eight breaths or work dynamically for eight rounds on each side.

CHAIR POSE TWIST 2

This utkatasana works a more open angle in the rotational axis. By using the lower arm against the leg, a pulling action similar to that of the twist allows for a more passive back bend than the first version of utkatasana. The leg that is being used as a lever has to abduct, helping to strengthen the muscles around the hip.

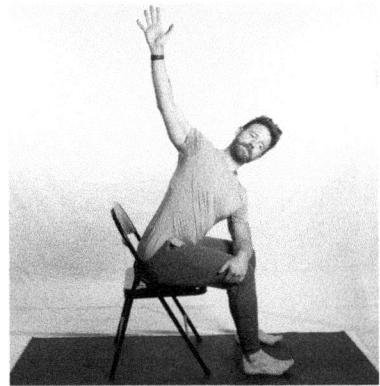

▶ In a parallel stance for the lower body, press down into active feet. Rest both elbows on the knees and lengthen the spine forwards away from the hips.

▶ Internally rotate the left arm to hold the outside of the right knee (or if that is too far, hold the left knee).

▶ Inhale to telescope the ribs forwards.

▶ Exhale to rotate the chest to the right, lifting the right arm.

▶ Hold for eight breaths and repeat on the other side.

CHAIR POSE TWIST 3

The stack of the arms in this pose allows for some really strong leverage into the rotation. The forearm bones need to be stacked in a straight line to access the lever; if the top arm folds back down towards the body, the thoracic rotation will be limited.

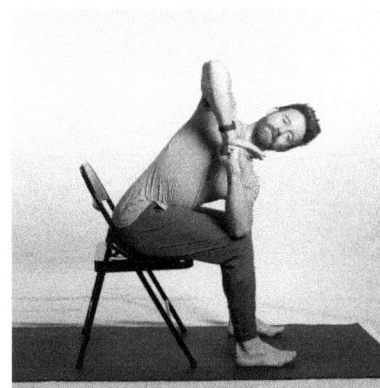

▶ In a parallel stance for the lower body, press down into active feet. Rest both elbows on the knees and lengthen the spine forwards away from the hips.

▶ Exhale to hook the left elbow outside of the right knee. If this is too challenging, either bring the feet closer together or rest the elbow to the inside of the left knee. Ball the left hand into a fist.

▶ Stack the right palm atop the left fist, keeping the wrist bones in line with the forearms.

▶ Inhale to lift the breastbone in line with the hands.

▶ Exhale to press down into the arms to rotate the chest to the right.

▶ Hold for eight breaths and repeat on the other side.

CHAIR POSE TWIST AT THE WALL

This variation of utkatasana is done with the front of the torso facing the wall. To change sides, the chair has to turn around 180 degrees, if you are able to do that. The wall allows for both arms to be involved in a pulling action, inviting the recruitment of more muscles in the upper back.

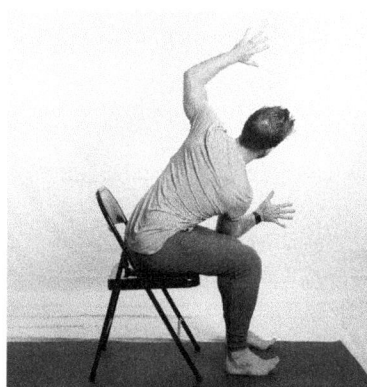

▶ Start with a chair placed one foot away from a wall with the left side facing the wall first. In a parallel stance for the lower body, press down into active feet. Rest both elbows on the knees and lengthen the spine forwards away from the hips.

▶ Exhale to hook the right elbow outside of the left knee, placing both hands onto the wall. If it is too challenging to maintain the elbow contact, hover the elbow above the legs with the hands on the wall.

▶ Inhale to lengthen the spine away from the pelvis.

▶ Exhale to turn the chest towards the wall, creating a pulling down action with the hands on the wall.

▶ Hold for eight breaths, turn the chair and repeat on the other side.

DYNAMIC TWIST

These twists are a firm favourite in my chair classes. The wider leg position allows for a greater forward bend, getting the axis of rotation almost parallel to the floor (without a block, it is usually parallel). Engaging more of the back muscles and core, these twists should be a daily staple to mobilise the spine.

▶ In a wider horse stance with the thighs wide and feet turned out, place a block on the floor in between the legs at a height that allows you to bend forwards comfortably with the hands on the block directly under the shoulders. Start with both hands on the block and lengthen the spine away from the hips.

▶ Inhale to rotate the chest to the right with the arm extended upwards.

▶ Exhale to return to centre and lengthen the spine.

▶ If the shoulder of the lifted arm isn't happy, cross the arm on the chest and do the rotations without the shoulder.

▶ Repeat this eight times on one side and then do the other side.

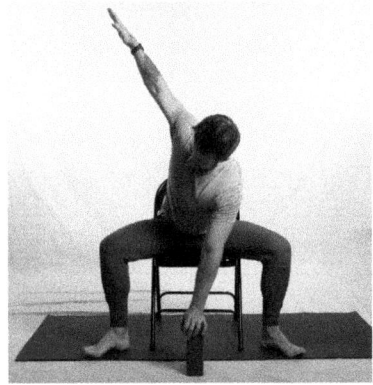

DYNAMIC TWIST WITH NECK ISOMETRICS

Adding weight to poses can help bring a bit of resistance training into your practice. By placing the hand on the back of the head and resisting the downward pressure with the neck and upper back, not only will the muscles have to work harder but the entire rotation will feel stronger and more aligned too.

▶ In a wider horse stance, with the thighs wide and feet turned out, place a block on

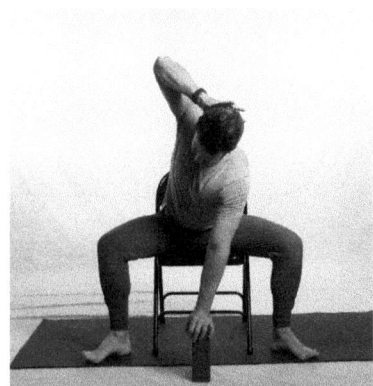

94

the floor in between the legs at a height that allows you to bend forward comfortably with the hands on the block directly under the shoulders. Start with both hands on the block and lengthen the spine away from the hips. Place the right hand onto the back of the head and press the head into the hand.

▶ Inhale to rotate the chest to the left, keeping the spine long.

▶ Exhale to return to centre and lengthen the spine.

▶ Repeat this eight times on one side and then do the other side.

TWISTING SQUAT 1

As mentioned at the start of this chapter, twists are really quite incredible at employing the other joints of the body. The blocks here allow for a deeper flex in the hips in a wider stance, very much like malasana, the yogi squat, or dead bug. Both legs have to press outwards to maintain the foundation while the spine rotates.

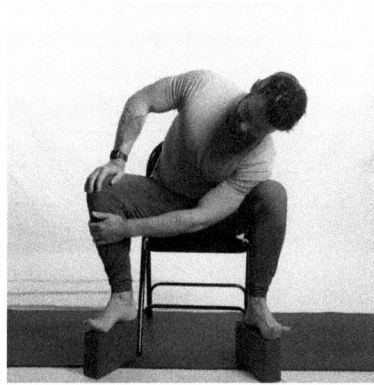

▶ Place both feet on blocks in the wider horse stance, with the thighs wide and feet turned out. Lean forwards between the legs.

▶ Lean the left side of your body against the left thigh, holding the right shin with the left hand. Place the right hand on top of the right thigh.

▶ Inhale to lengthen the spine towards the left knee, twisting on a diagonal.

▶ Exhale to press with the right arm to turn the chest and pull with the left hand.

▶ Hold for eight breaths and repeat on the other side.

TWISTING SQUAT 2

Much like in the dynamic twist, extending the arm in this pose can add a lot to the upper back. The first stage of this pose may need to be repeated several times. Given that the axis of rotation veers off on a diagonal, the extending arm can assist in creating the feeling of space on the same side of the body.

▶ Place both feet on blocks in the wider horse stance. Lean forwards between the legs.

▶ Lean the left side of your body against the left thigh, holding the right shin with the left hand.

▶ Inhale to lengthen the spine towards the left knee, twisting on a diagonal.

▶ Exhale to pull with the left hand, reaching the right hand upwards, drawing the shoulder blade back towards the spine.

▶ Hold for eight breaths and repeat on the other side.

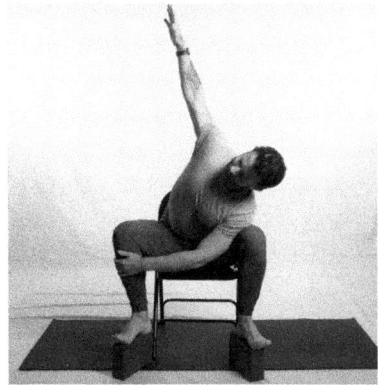

TWISTING LUNGE

Commanding strength and support through the lower body, this twist is one of stability and control. It allows the practitioner to feel the duality between open and closed joints, with the possibility of removing the block to change the rotational axis. Deep breathing will bring this pose to life in an incredible way.

▶ From seated, place the left thigh and sit bone on the chair and send the right leg off to the side straight. Place a block to the inside of the left ankle.

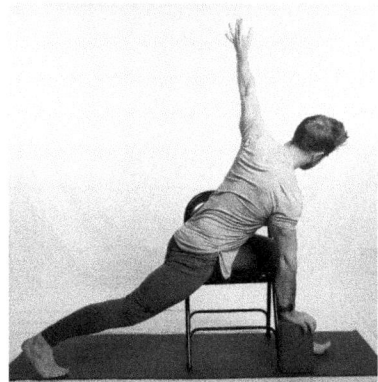

- ▶ Turning the torso towards the left leg, place the right hand onto the block, resting the left hand onto the left thigh. Pivot up onto the toes of the right leg to level the hips.

- ▶ Inhale to twist towards the left leg and reach the left arm upwards.

- ▶ Exhale to stick your butt out, drawing the shoulder blades down the back.

- ▶ Hold for eight breaths and repeat on the other side.

TWISTING TRIANGLE

This is a twist, a forward bend, a hamstring lengthener and a spinal extension conditioner all in one. With so many parts, it can be really challenging. If it feels like it is too much, build up by doing some of the hip opening twists and forward bends from previous chapters for a while.

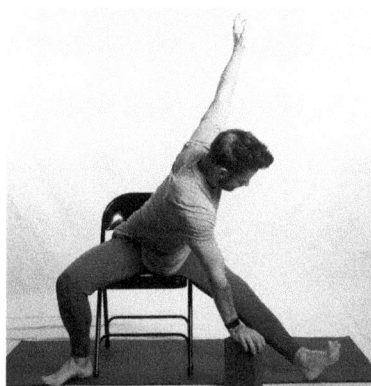

- ▶ In a wider stance, like horse, straighten the left leg out, either resting on the heel as pictured or with the foot flat. Place a block to the inside of this leg.

- ▶ Place the right hand on the block.

- ▶ Inhale to lengthen the torso towards the left knee.

- ▶ Exhale to rotate towards the left leg, reaching the left arm upwards.

- ▶ Hold for eight breaths and repeat on the other side.

CHAPTER EIGHT

STANDING POSES

A lot of the poses we have been working with so far use fairly symmetrical lower body foundations, but to really increase the vocabulary of poses, adding in more elements, like recruiting the lower body in different ways, is key. The following poses are classed as standing poses; using a chair creates a gateway into exploring the sensations and attributes of these poses. Poses like warriors and lunges can all be practised in a chair, and for the ease of indexing, we will use the names of the standing poses. If you attend a class or want to integrate your chair poses into a class, letting the teacher know that you know variations of standing poses will be helpful for both you and them.

In Forrest Yoga practices, the longer holds of standing poses usually come after warming up, core work and sun salutations, with a few linked together into a standing pose series. This means that similar muscles and movements are held in tension for 8–30 breaths. It is the long holds that allow the recruitment of slow-twitch muscle fibres as opposed to faster, more explosive strength. When moving from pose to pose, aiming to stay engaged and moving with care allows the tension to remain in the lower body.

Standing poses keep the spine in a relatively neutral position, with less demand on the back and postural muscles. In this neutral position, forces are directed to the limbs. When the impulse from the legs is transferred into the pelvis, and into the spine, pressure can be taken off the spine. In this way, the spine is supported in flexion (forward bending), extension (backward bending), rotation (twisting) and lateral flexion (side bending), with some poses combining some of these actions. Building a foundation from the ground up creates a multi-faceted awareness and helps integrate the muscular engagements without focusing on balancing.

In this section, there are some poses in which you are invited to explore balancing with the aid of the chair. Poses where we balance on one leg encourage the automatic engagement of muscles that support the hip, like the TFL and gluteus minimus. Over time, strengthening these muscles can help stabilise the hips and lower back. In particular, to help build strength in the quadratus lumborum (QL), over stretching can be detrimental. In poses like triangle, the QL can engage to support the spine horizontal to the floor, encouraging extra engagement from the obliques.

Some of the poses in Chapter Seven on twisting and Chapter Five on forward bending could easily be included in this chapter, but when we get to the sample sequences, they will come together without having to repeat the same information.

> At the age of 50 I fractured the femur on my amputated leg. After having a pin inserted, I was discharged from hospital with a pair of crutches but no referral to physio. By the time I was able to wear a prosthetic again, the thigh muscles had atrophied and I had to use two sticks to help me walk. After several years of struggling, I became aware of a yoga teacher offering chair yoga for amputees. From my first lesson, I never looked back. My balance and core strength improved enormously, which allowed me to walk without the aid of sticks. It is not an exaggeration to say it gave me my life back. So much so that when I again fractured my femur a second time at the age of 73, chair yoga was instrumental in my recovery from the beginning by building core muscle strength and flexible joints.
>
> *Ella*

SIDE BEND IN HORSE

Activating the lower body in a symmetrical position can help to support the lower back. This also serves as the postural foundation for many of the warrior arm positions if moving the legs towards straight isn't yet possible. Feel free to use this lower body variation for warrior 2, reverse warrior, extended warrior and triangle.

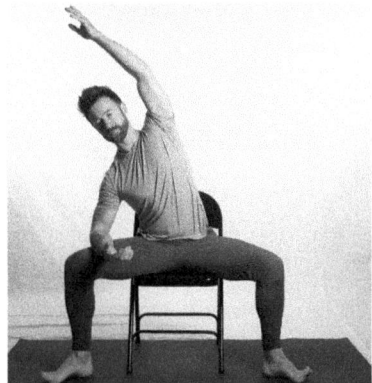

▶ In a wide stance, lean back against the chair to support the middle back.

▶ Inhale to telescope the ribs up.

▶ Exhale to side bend to the right, placing the right forearm on the right thigh. The left arm reaches overhead.

▶ Press down into active feet.

▶ Hold for eight breaths and repeat on the other side.

WARRIOR 2

The origin of the warrior poses comes from a tale of two warriors born from cracks in the ground rather than them being poses that are conducive to battle. The actions in the lower body symbolise the action of pulling apart, with the torso rising triumphantly from the split. They make for wonderful poses to build strength in the lower body and a lightness in the upper body.

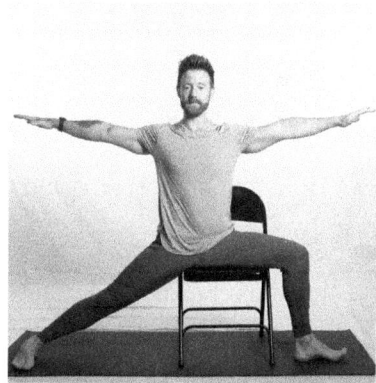

▶ Start in horse and slide to the right until the right thigh bone is clear of the seat of the chair.

▶ Turn the left foot to the left and set the right foot perpendicular to the right.

▶ Inhale to telescope the ribs up and extend the arms out at shoulder height.

▶ Exhale to press down into active feet and create a pressing away action with the legs.

▶ Hold for eight breaths and repeat on the other side.

REVERSE WARRIOR

Much like the side bend in horse, this allows for a side bend with a level pelvis in a warrior 2 stance. The asymmetry in the muscle activities of the hips creates an opportunity to access tight parts of the lower back in a way that the side bend in horse misses.

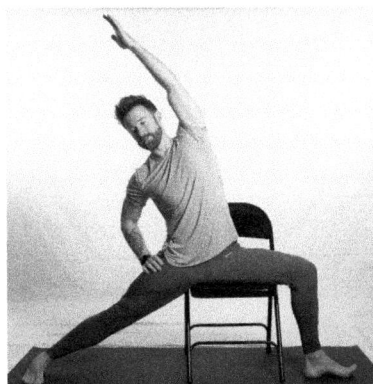

- ▶ From warrior 2, place the right hand on the right hip.

- ▶ Inhale to telescope the ribs up, lifting out of the lower back. Lift the left arm.

- ▶ Exhale to side bend over the right arm, drawing the shoulder blade down and wrap the left shoulder blade towards the chest.

- ▶ Hold for eight breaths and repeat on the other side.

- ▶ Over time the right hand may move further down the leg but avoid placing the hand on the knee.

EXTENDED WARRIOR

Different to reverse warrior, side bending over a flexed hip and opening up the opposite side of the back can create an exceptionally supported position for the lower back. Although not pictured, placing a block to the inside of the right leg can allow a little more depth to be found in the lateral flexion.

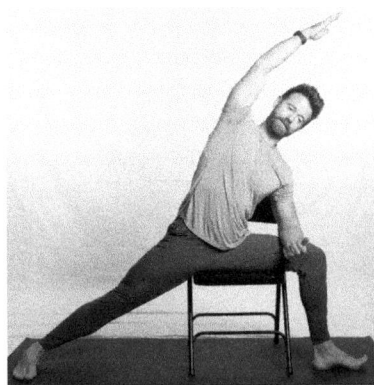

- ▶ From warrior 2, place the left forearm on the left thigh with the palm up.

- ▶ Inhale to lift the right arm overhead.

▶ Exhale to wrap the right shoulder blade towards the chest. Keep the neck relaxed.

▶ Hold for eight breaths and repeat on the other side.

HIGH LUNGE/WARRIOR 1

Warrior 2 poses occupy a realm of side bending and coronal plane movements. Moving into the sagittal plane, front facing, can be more challenging in a chair but is well worth exploring for a diverse range of actions and forces in the hips. Different to the lunges, these poses are more active in the legs and a bit longer in length.

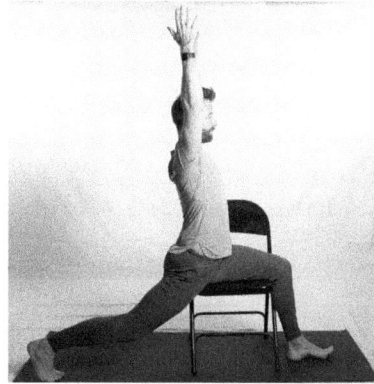

▶ Start in horse and slide to the right until the right thighbone is clear of the seat of the chair.

▶ Turn the left foot to the left and flip up onto the toes of the right leg (warrior 1 is conventionally taught with the heel down and the foot at quite a steep angle but this puts a lot of pressure on the ankle, knee, hips and back).

▶ Inhale to lift the arms up, squaring the chest and hips towards the left leg.

▶ Exhale to tuck your tailbone down, pressing down into both active feet.

▶ If the balance is challenging, ensure the feet are on two parallel lines about one foot apart and feel free to use an arm on the backrest of the chair.

▶ Hold for eight breaths and repeat on the other side.

TWISTING WARRIOR

This is one of my favourite poses when I feel like my back needs to be re-energised or is stiff. The chair supports a level pelvis, allowing for a deep twist in the mid and upper back while creating strength in the rear support leg.

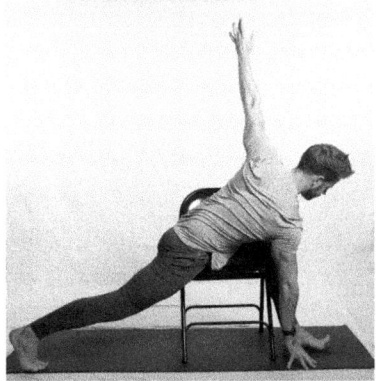

▶ Starting in high lunge/warrior 1, lean forwards onto the left leg. Bring the right hand down to the floor or a block.

▶ Inhale to lengthen the spine towards the left knee and stick your butt out.

▶ Exhale to rotate towards the left leg, reaching the left hand upwards.

▶ Hold for eight breaths and repeat on the other side.

TRIANGLE

The triangle standing pose usually has two straight legs, but when seated, find a way to place yourself in the chair so that the front leg is given preference so it can be straight. Given that the rear leg and top arm contribute very little to the overall structure of the standing pose, emphasis will be placed here on the straight leg and lower arm. The lateral flexion, core work and hamstring stretch can all be felt one side at a time.

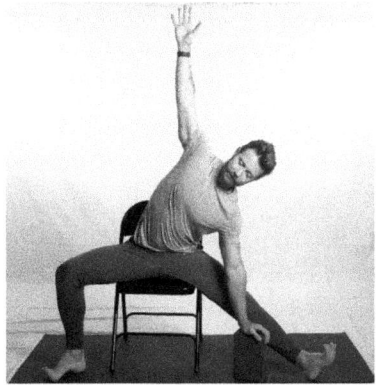

▶ From horse, straighten the left leg in the same angle. The left foot can be flat or flexed like the image.

▶ Inhale to telescope the ribs up.

▶ Exhale to draw the left thighbone towards the pelvis, creating a slight lift on the right sit bone and lean over the left leg. Place the left hand on a block by the left shin and lift the right arm above.

▶ Lengthen the spine away from the pelvis, aiming to keep both sides of the abdomen long.

▶ Hold for eight breaths and repeat on the other side.

KNEE TO CHEST

Pulling the knee into the chest not only allows for a bit of abdominal pressure but also flexes the hip. The aim is to keep the pelvis still so that the lower back is not contributing to the movement, dissociating flexing the hip from flexing the spine. Using abdominal breathing with compression also tightens the thoracolumbar fascia, thus lifting the torso and supporting the lumbar spine.

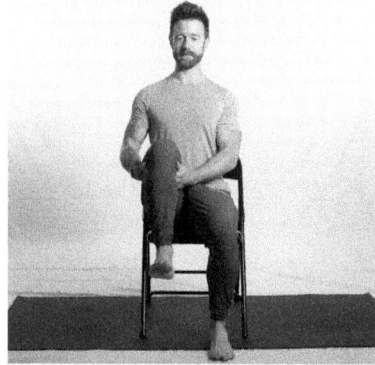

▶ Sit back against the frame of the chair and lengthen the spine upwards.

▶ Exhale to pick up the right thigh, drawing it into the chest without moving the lower back.

▶ Take eight deep abdominal breaths here and repeat on the other side.

BACK RELEASE

Knee to chest pose will show you whether you will be able to cross the foot of the lifted leg over the opposite thigh. If you can't yet, moving closer to the front of the chair will allow the thigh bone of the other leg to be at a lower angle and can assist with the cross.

▶ From knee to chest pose, with the left leg to the chest, cross the left ankle over the right thigh just above the knee. Make sure the contact point is at the lower leg bones of the left leg rather than bending the ankle joint itself.

▶ Inhale to telescope the ribs up.

▶ Exhale to widen the left thigh, flexing the left foot and sticking the butt out.

▶ If the pose is feeling accessible, lean forwards without rounding the back.

▶ Hold for eight breaths and repeat on the other side.

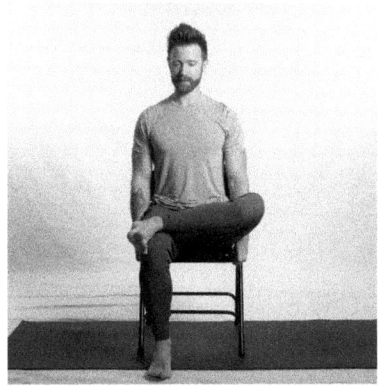

LUNGE HEEL TO BUTT

This pose has numerous points of contact, but as it shifts from the lunge position, it actually turns into a balance. The rewards are worth the logistical challenge of getting into the pose. Tight quads put a lot of pressure into the joints both above and below the thigh, making this an important muscle group to access. If you need more lift (notice that two blocks are used in the image), stack up however many blocks you need to get a solid balance point.

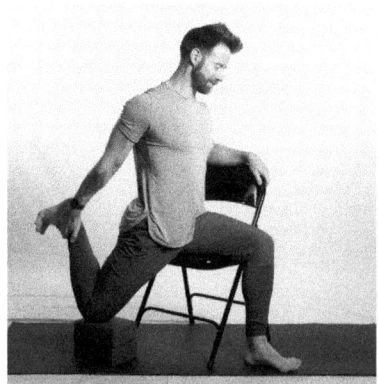

▶ Start in high lunge/warrior 1 and set the right knee on a block or stack of blocks. Use the left hand to hold the backrest of the chair.

▶ Exhale to reach the right arm down towards the right ankle as you bend the leg. If you cannot grab the ankle, use a strap or towel.

▶ Inhale to telescope the ribs up.

▶ Exhale to tuck your tailbone down to increase the stretch on the quads.

▶ Hold for eight breaths and repeat on the other side.

LUNGE SIDE BEND

Like the previous lunge, this pose can be done with or without blocks under the knee. Without blocks, the ability to reach down with the thigh bone allows for a deeper stretch into the side body, creating a strong stretch into the abdomen, side wall of the abdomen, hip flexors and quad.

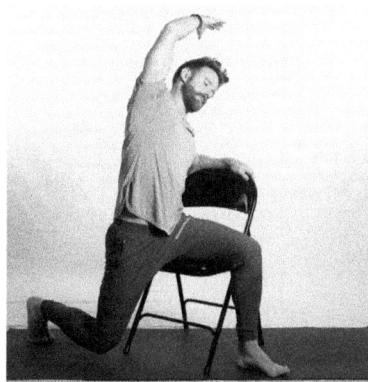

▶ Start in high lunge/warrior 1 and set the right knee on a block or stack of blocks.

▶ Inhale to lift the right arm up, telescoping the ribs up.

▶ Exhale to side bend to the left and tuck the tailbone down. Use a strong pulling in of the abdominal muscles with each exhale.

▶ Hold for eight breaths and repeat on the other side.

CHAIR-ASSISTED ANKLE STRENGTHENER 1

Building strength and support below the knee is also very important for standing poses. Using a chair or a countertop, these two movements will challenge your thighs, calves and feet to build endurance for balancing. This action is linked to the next image – to work both of them together.

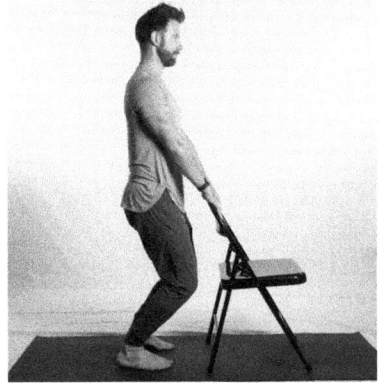

▶ Stand facing the rear of the chair, with the feet parallel so that when the legs bend the knees are going straight forwards over the toes.

▶ Keeping the feet flat, inhale to bend the legs; the chest stays upright.

CHAIR-ASSISTED ANKLE STRENGTHENER 2

▶ Starting from chair-assisted ankle strengthener 1, exhale to lift to the tiptoes, keeping the legs bent.

▶ Inhale to slowly lower the heels down, keeping the legs bent.

▶ Repeat ten times and then straighten the legs.

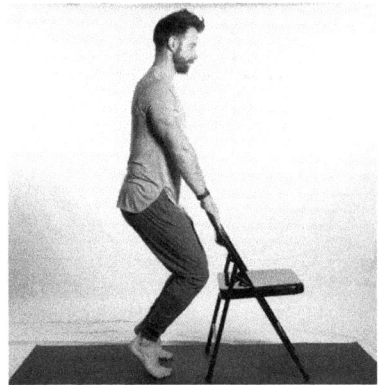

SINGLE LEG BALANCE

So far, our standing poses have remained fairly connected to the ground. To augment the passive hip flex of knee to chest pose, we can experiment with both balance and hip flexion in this exercise.

▶ Facing the chair, place both hands on the seat so the hands are under the shoulders. Step the feet back until in a plank position with the body in a straight line from the feet to the shoulders.

▶ Shift the weight onto your left foot and squeeze the left thigh bone to the right to engage the hip stabilisers.

▶ Exhale to bring the right foot off the floor and bring the right knee under the hips towards the abdomen.

▶ Inhale to set the right leg back.

▶ Alternate sides slowly until you have done six rounds.

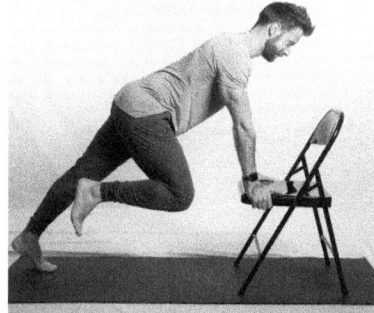

WARRIOR 3

Thinking of the warrior poses as a ranking isn't a great way to look at them; each offers something quite different, but it does just so happen that warrior 3 feels like the strongest pose due to the emphasis on the standing leg. It is a great opportunity to strengthen the hamstrings, butt muscles and erector muscles while remaining well balanced using the chair.

▶ Standing in front of the chair, place both hands on the seat so the hands are under the shoulders and the feet are under the hips.

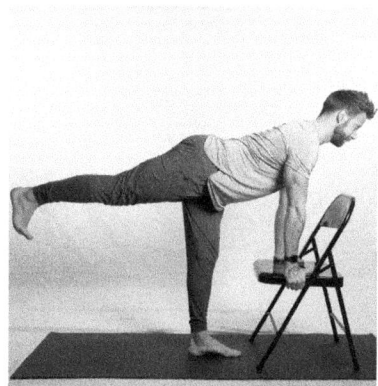

- ▶ Shift the weight into the left foot and squeeze the left thigh bone to the right to switch on the muscles of the hip.

- ▶ Inhale to telescope the ribs forwards and push down into the hands, look slightly forwards.

- ▶ Exhale to shift the right leg straight back maintaining a long flat back.

- ▶ Hold for eight breaths and repeat on the other side.

HALF MOON

Using the flexibility of triangle for the hamstrings, this pose presents rotation and balance challenges. The pose can be entered in a couple of different ways – from rotating open from warrior 3 (if the hip will allow it) to setting up with the legs bent side on and leaning into the chair.

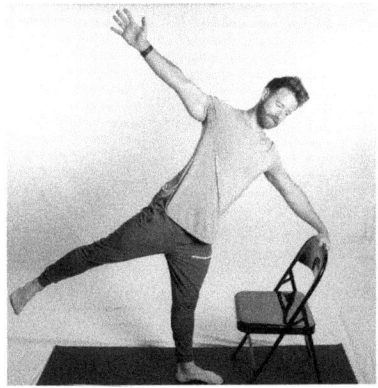

- ▶ Place the feet a few inches away from the chair, with the toes pointing towards the chair. Set the left hand onto the backrest of the chair.

- ▶ Inhale to shift the weight onto the left foot and left hand.

- ▶ Exhale to flex the right foot, lifting the thigh until the outer hip muscles kick in.

- ▶ Hold for eight breaths and repeat on the other side.

TREE

This is a more challenging balance, with the weight fully off the hands. The balance can be steadied by placing support under the rotated thigh, but it will take some refinement using a block or two, or even a towel, to get the height just right. In the balance, feel for the small movements and shifts rather than stillness.

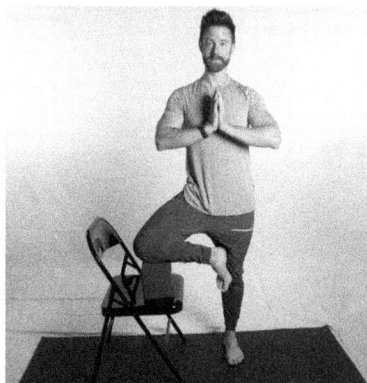

▶ Standing to the side of the chair with the right thigh closest to it, place a block on the seat. Shift the weight onto the left leg and engage the inner thigh of the left leg by squeezing the left thighbone to the right.

▶ With the arms relaxed, begin to lift the right leg, setting the knee/shin on the blocks. The right foot can rest on the inner left thigh.

▶ The hands can rest on the hips or together at the heart.

▶ Hold for eight breaths and then repeat on the other side.

CHAPTER NINE

DYNAMIC MOVEMENT

In the chair classes I teach, I like people to get grounded in the basics and create movement in some of the sticky places before adding in dynamic movement or sequences. Once people have explored all the parts that make up a sequence, I take time to build their familiarity and stamina through an increasing number of repetitions. The sequences here are based around surya namaskar, sun salutations, and while they are often seen as a warm-up, I like them to be in the meaty bit of practice, as well as to warm up for them in advance.

Sun salutations consist of lengthening and strengthening, forward bends and back bends in sequence that engage various muscles. The coordination of breath and movement can help with respiratory issues, concentration and cardiovascular health. Along with the physical benefits they provide, moving sequences don't leave room for much else in your head, so their ability to cultivate a deeper connection shouldn't be minimised.

Once sun salutations are part of your practice, you can really diversify your daily sessions by varying the number of repetitions, pausing in certain poses for a few breaths and adding in poses like back bends or twists (some examples will be given). As there are no set rules, you may even end up creating a salutation that gives you everything you need, and it will be like meeting a good friend every day.

Over time, you may start to realise that your sun salutations are very much in the front-to-back sagittal plane of movement. This isn't a problem, especially if these movement patterns don't occur often in your day-to-day life, but adding in things like side bends after the first reach up will allow for that.

Personally, after sun salutations, I feel like my body is ready for anything, and adding in back bends or standing pose variations will do wonders for increasing the movement vocabulary.

If you are teaching these dynamic movements, it is helpful to first demonstrate the sequence at pace with some instructions and observations and then do one round spending a little more time in each pose. Then, usually with the reassurance of 'don't panic', explain that you are going to move with the breath through the sequence.

SUN SALUTATION A

Consisting of forward bends, spinal extension and hip hinges, this seated salutation is a great way to integrate the various ways you can move your spine and posterior chain.

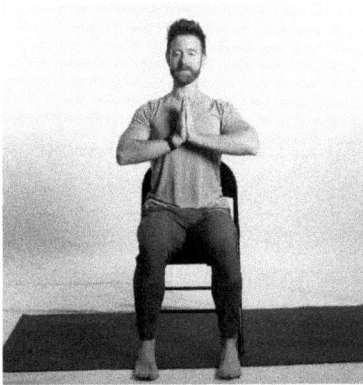

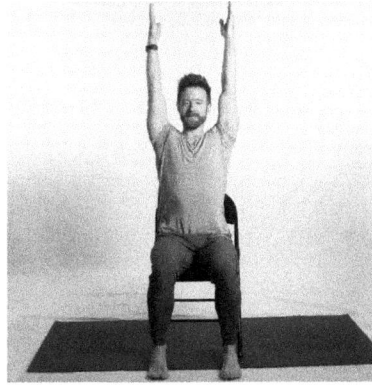

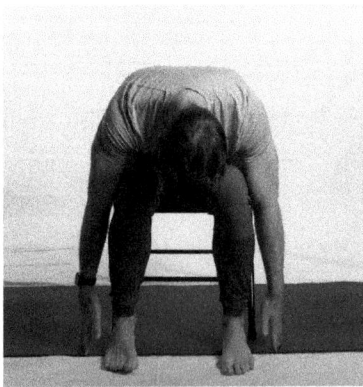

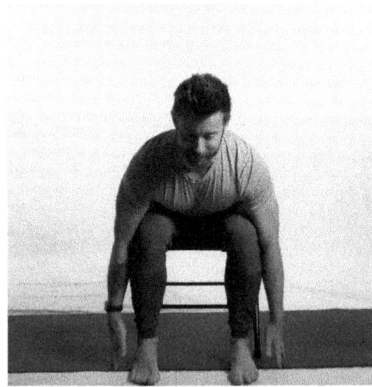

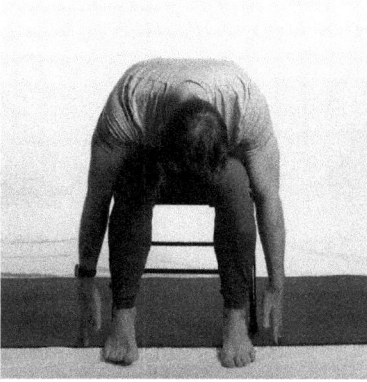
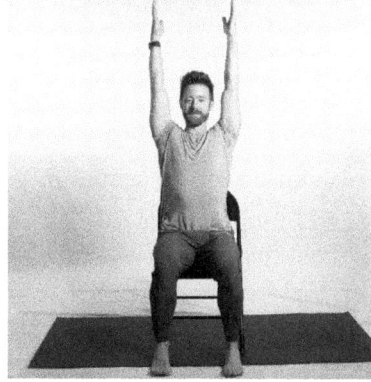

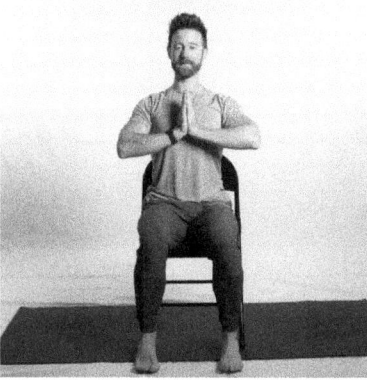

▶ Start seated with the hands together at the chest.

▶ Inhale to reach the arms up.

▶ Exhale into a forward bend (feel free to use blocks set outside of the feet to set the hands onto).

▶ Inhale into a halfway lift, lengthening the skull forwards.

▶ Exhale into a forward bend.

▶ Inhale to scoop the chest forwards and up to seated with the arms up.

▶ Exhale to bring the hands together at the chest.

CLASSICAL SUN SALUTATION

This salutation involves a bit more of the deadlift-like action of coming up to seated a few times to bring the knees into the chest. With the additional hip flexion, this salutation can be wonderful for a tight lower back and to do before back bending and standing poses.

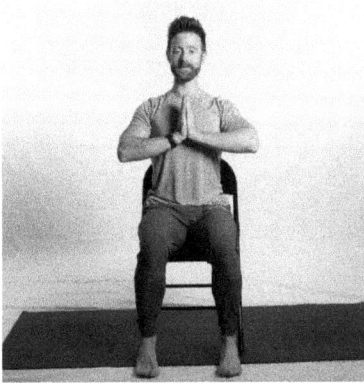

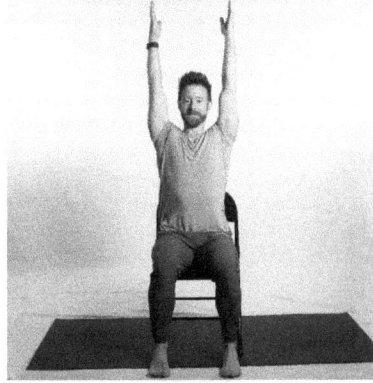

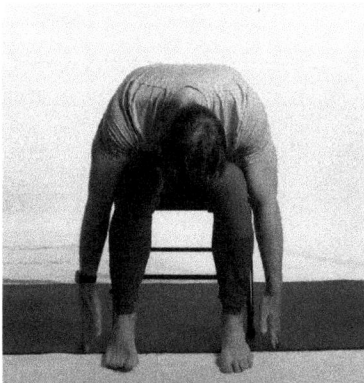

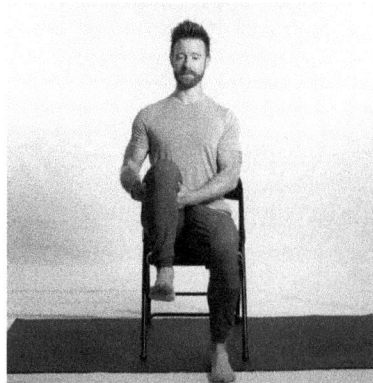

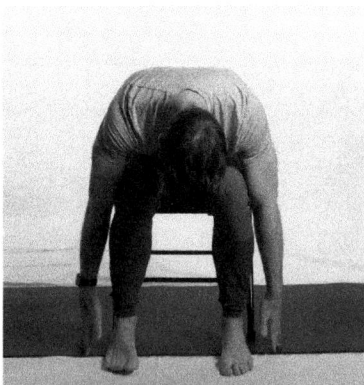

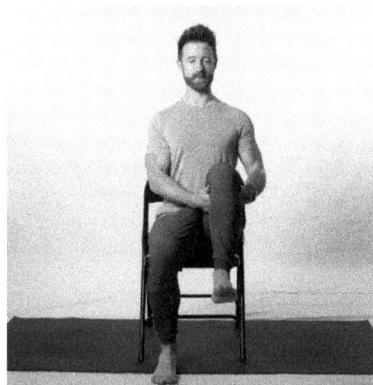

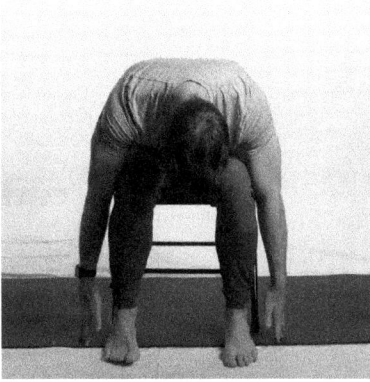

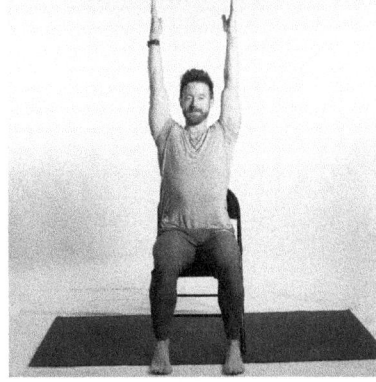

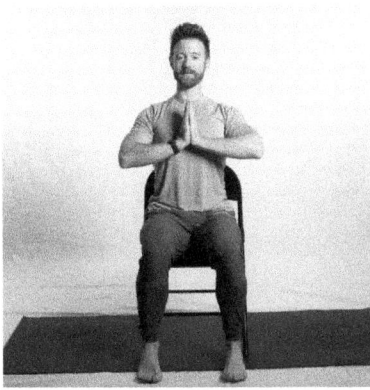

- ▶ Start seated with the hands together at the chest.

- ▶ Inhale to reach the arms up.

- ▶ Exhale into a forward bend (feel free to use blocks for the hands).

- ▶ Inhale to lift up to seated, bringing the right knee into the chest.

- ▶ Exhale into a forward bend.

- ▶ Inhale to lift up to seated, bringing the left knee into the chest.

- ▶ Exhale into a forward bend.

- ▶ Inhale to scoop the chest forwards and up to seated with the arms up.

- ▶ Exhale to bring the hands together at the chest.

SUN SALUTATION A (VARIATION)

This sun salutation adds in twisting poses to the start of the sequence, which could easily be replaced with back bends or side bends to give variety to the movements you are doing. In classes with more experienced practitioners, we do a few regular sun salutation As and a couple with twists and a couple with back bends to get the heart rate up.

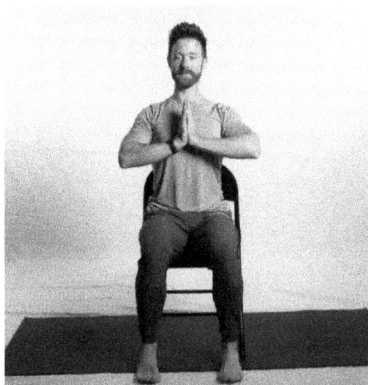

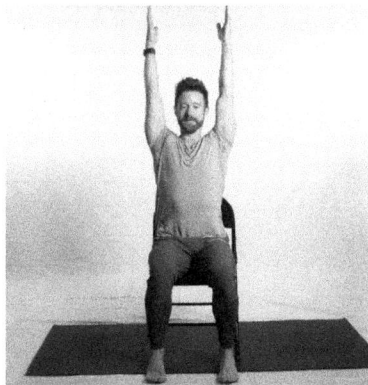

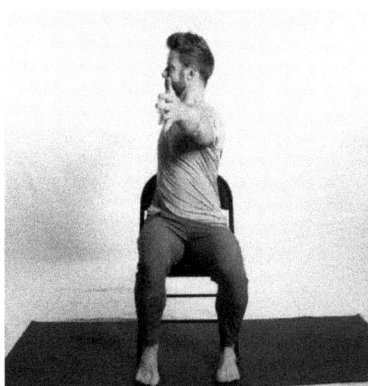

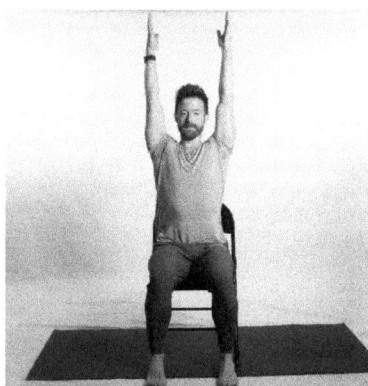

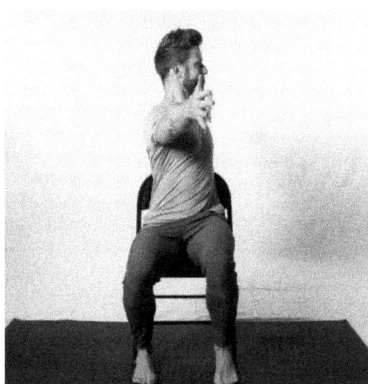

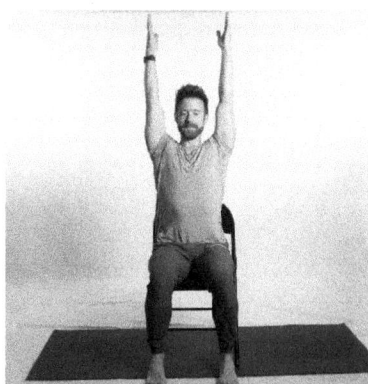

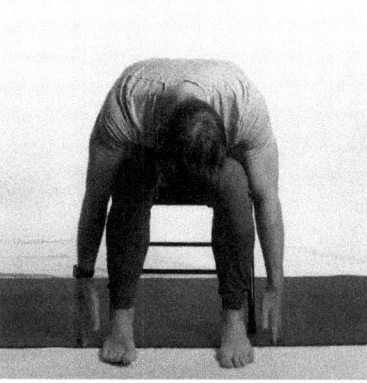

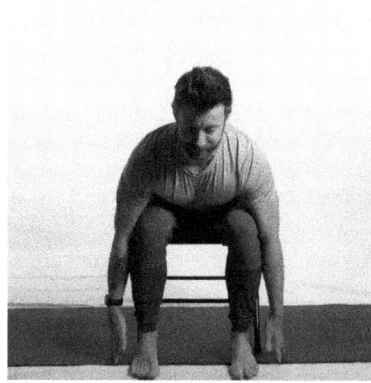

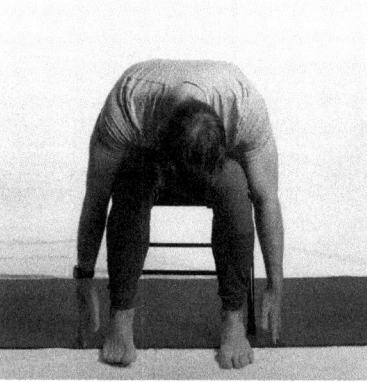

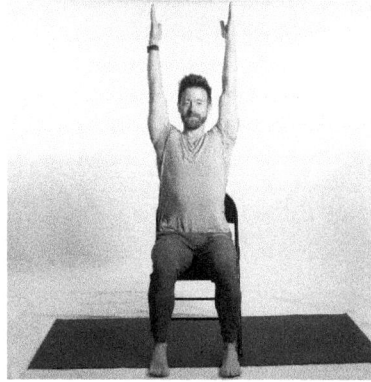

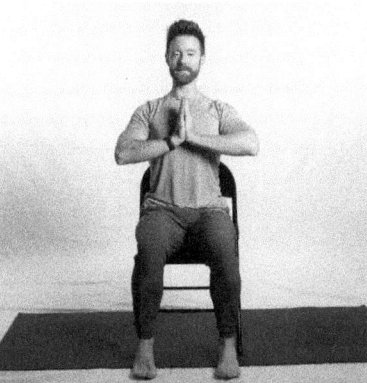

- ▶ Start seated with the hands together at the chest.

- ▶ Inhale to reach the arms up.

- ▶ Exhale to twist to the right with the arms out wide.

- ▶ Inhale to reach the arms up.

- ▶ Exhale to twist to the left with the arms out wide.

- ▶ Inhale to reach the arms up.

- ▶ Exhale into a forward bend (feel free to use blocks for the hands).

- ▶ Inhale into a halfway lift, lengthening the skull forwards.

- ▶ Exhale into a forward bend.

- ▶ Inhale to scoop the chest forwards and up to seated with the arms up.

- ▶ Exhale to bring the hands together at the chest.

SUN SALUTATION B

This sequence uses utkatasana to add in more dynamic movement. With extra movement for the shoulders and of a back bending nature, this is a great complement to a back bending practice.

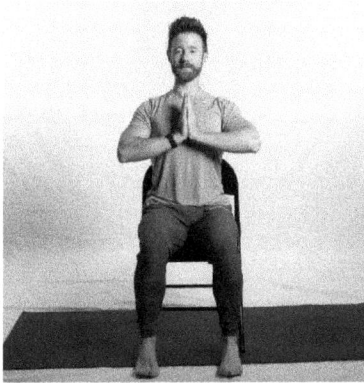

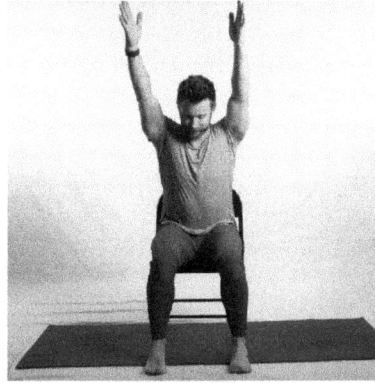

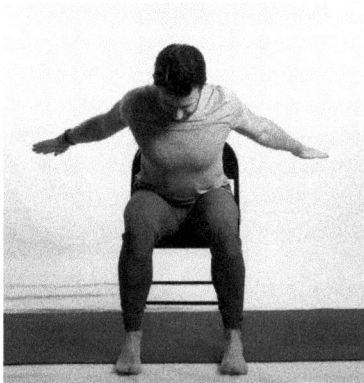

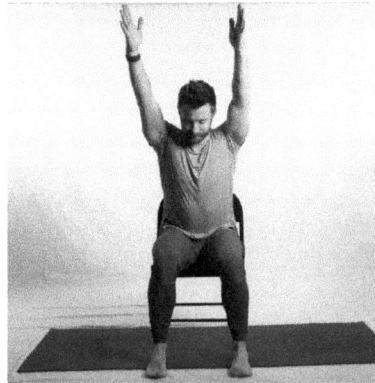

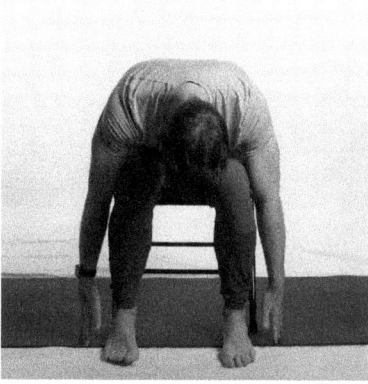
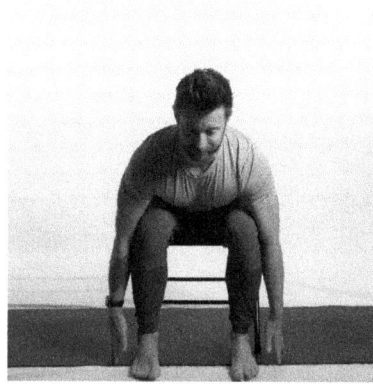

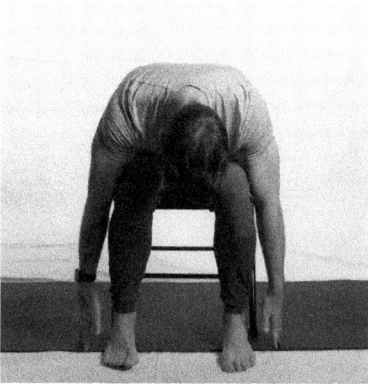
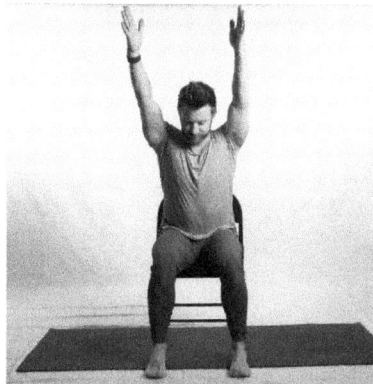

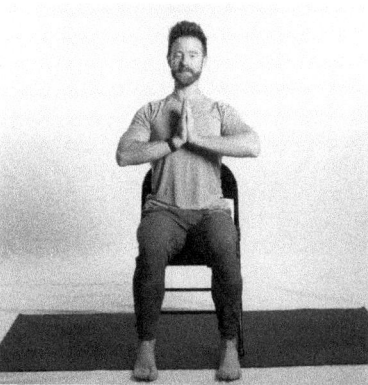

- ▶ Start seated with the hands together at the chest.

- ▶ Inhale to reach the arms up into utkatasana.

- ▶ Exhale to sweep the arms back into airplane arms.

- ▶ Inhale to reach the arms and chest forwards into utkatasana.

- ▶ Exhale into a forward bend (feel free to use blocks for the hands).

▶ Inhale into a halfway lift, lengthening the skull forwards.

▶ Exhale into a forward bend.

▶ Inhale to scoop the chest forwards and up to utkatasana.

▶ Exhale to bring the hands together at the chest.

HIP CIRCUMDUCTION

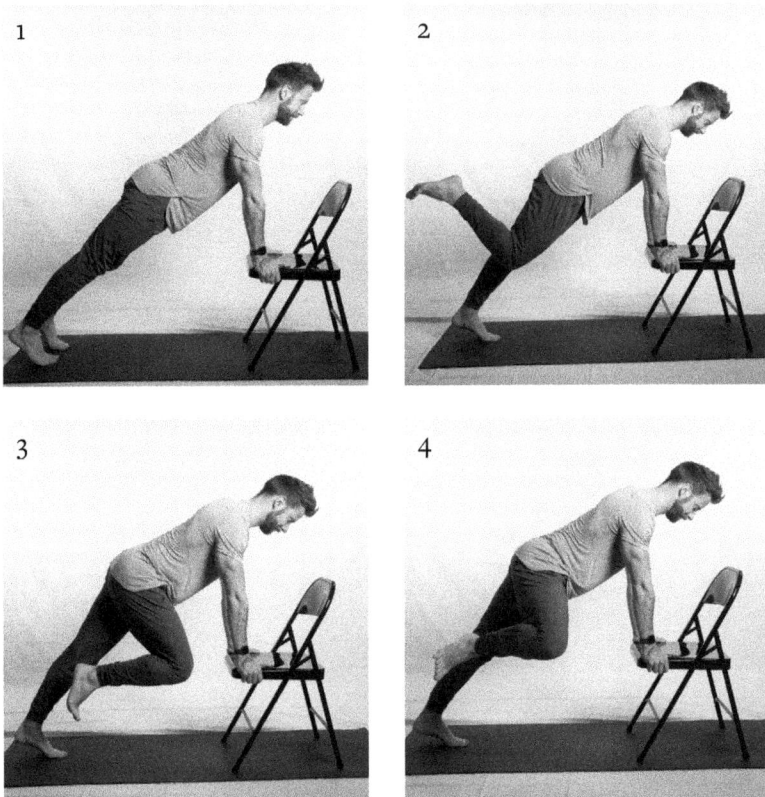

One of the things I get people to explore in classes is their relationship to their hips. A lot of the time, we end up being strong in one or two movements but miss a lot of the other aspects or adapt into habits like moving the entire pelvis and lower spine to move the leg. This sequence, with the stabilisation of the chair, allows for the various actions of the hip to be explored while keeping the pelvis totally still. Over time, this will start to feel easier and will give you greater familiarity with your own range of motion. This sequence also makes for a wonderful (albeit a strong) warm-up for standing poses.

▶ Start in a plank position, holding the seat of the chair, with the elbows straight and the feet hip distance apart. If balance is a challenge, stack the feet directly under the hips (1).

▶ Start by bending the right leg 90 degrees while keeping the thigh bones in line with each other (2).

▶ Exhale to flex the hip, bringing the right knee towards the chest (3).

▶ Inhale to open the right knee out to the right without moving the pelvis (4).

▶ Exhale to drive the leg back, internally rotating the thigh, with the 90-degree bend in line with the opposite thigh (2).

▶ Inhale to place the foot down (1).

▶ Repeat this circle of movement in the opposite direction (crossing the right leg to the left, under the left hip, and back).

▶ Do three of each direction and then repeat on the other side.

CHAPTER TEN

RELAXING

Modern life is stressful. The body is stimulated from every direction, both physically and mentally, and our yoga practice can be a bastion against a state of chronic stress. Breathing practices, restorative poses and the final relaxation pose (savasana) aim to recalibrate the nervous system by allowing practitioners to fully relax, releasing tensions in the body and the mind.

This can shift the nervous system from a state of sympathetic dominance towards the rest-and-digest mode of the autonomic nervous system, reducing the production of stress hormones like cortisol. As we practise, the body is working with awareness of the increasingly subtle, and as our practice warms down, we move towards a steady heart rate and calm breath. This downregulated nervous system supports our digestive system, mood and sleep.

This part of our practice, especially outside of a led class, is often skipped, as we can be hardwired to feel like we need to be upregulated, busy and productive. So, as much as it may be challenging, I encourage you to stick around for this part.

During restorative poses or relaxation, the focus isn't on doing but instead is on being. Initially, it can be useful to simply observe yourself breathing – not changing it, simply observing. Eventually, this may become observing thoughts, feelings and sensations in the body. Unlike other relaxing activities that involve doing something, like walking, or cooking, here, we are instead looking to reduce the external stimulation and look within.

In yoga philosophy (specifically the path set out in the Yoga Sutras of Patanjali), there is a concept called pratyahara, sensory withdrawal, that precedes concentration and then meditation. Before trying to meditate, the Sutras say, we need to reduce the external stimulus and cultivate focus. During these poses, there should be very little to no stretch; instead, there should be a fully supported and relaxed form with a natural flow of breath. Sensory withdrawal can be as simple as closing the eyes, switching off the music or TV, wrapping up in a blanket so the body is comfortable and observing your breathing.

As you meet the poses in this section, you can either put a few into a restorative sequence or choose different versions as part of your cool-down, but do take the time at the end of your practice to integrate all that you have done – to enjoy a moment of calm. You may feel your hands and feet getting cold and your stomach rumbling – that means you made it! Your body moved into a rest-and-digest state! Personally, when I am not in a class, there is a chance I might drift off, so I usually set a timer to give myself five to ten minutes in silent contemplation. For extra comfort, feel free to move to the couch to lie down fully so the front of the hips feel more open.

RESTORATIVE SINGLE LEG FORWARD BEND

Using this pose not as a final relaxation pose but to support in a relaxed way for a few minutes can bring great change to the tone of the muscles on the back of the body. In the picture, the foot is elevated on a bolster and chair, but even a folded blanket – something to take away the distraction of the hardness of the chair – would be good.

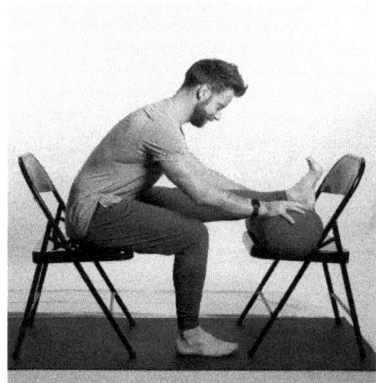

Once the arms are resting either on the second chair, or on the thigh, aim to be in restorative single forward bend pose for two minutes and then repeat on the other side.

SAVASANA

Leaning back against the chair and slightly elevating the feet will allow the postural heavy lifters to switch off, especially around the hips and the lower back. With the hands resting in the lap, awareness can be brought to the passive movement of the breath. Savasana poses can be held for a few minutes at the end of practice – the longer the practice, the longer the savasana.

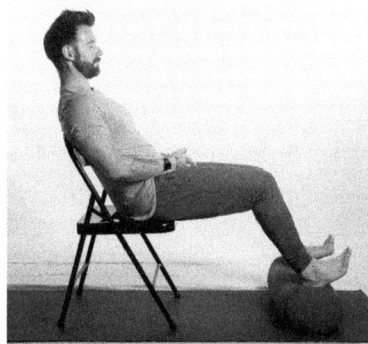

CHEST OPENER SAVASANA

This can be done with the hands resting in the lap or down by the side. The bolster or rolled up towel or mat is placed between the spine and the chair to provide some support for the spine. Setting the chair near a wall will also allow the head and neck to be supported.

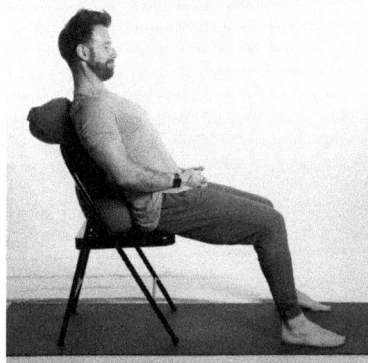

LEGS UP SAVASANA

Allowing the weight to shift into the pelvis by elevating the legs can make for a great rest position. To further support the pose, having the chair that is being sat on near the wall so the head can rest against something can be useful. If you don't have a bolster, a pillow will work well.

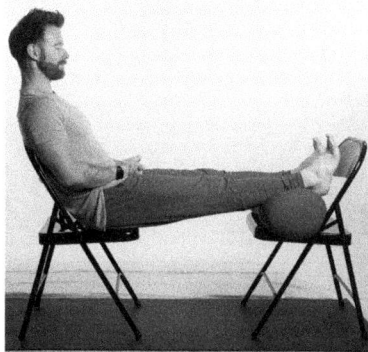

SUPPORTED FORWARD BEND

To take the pressure off the back of the body, and to allow the muscles that support the head and neck to relax, this pose is a treat.

Start with the feet wider than hip distance apart or in a relaxed horse stance. Lean forwards onto the bolster so that the weight of the crossed hands, head and torso is supported. Placing a blanket between the hands and head can also support the neck if the reach is too far.

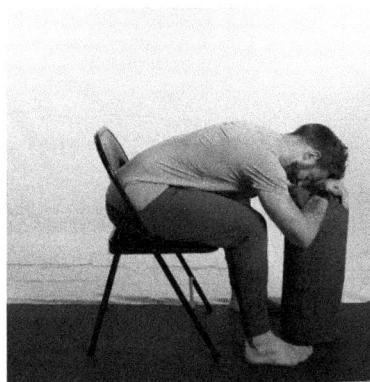

DELUXE SAVASANA

Now, this does look busy but it is incredible. Working with horse stance, if that keeps the hips relaxed, you can elevate the feet on blocks to create a bit more hip opening. Using a second chair and a bolster, pull them in close until you can rest your torso and head onto the bolster. This can also be done with both legs wide and straight.

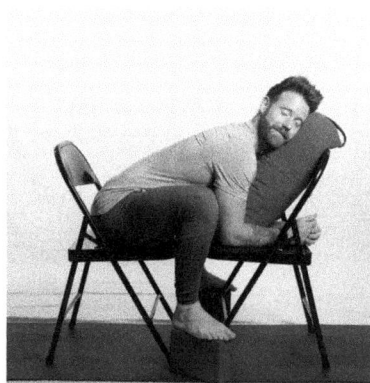

CHAPTER ELEVEN

BREATHWORK

Breathing is an essential function that runs automatically from birth. It is unique because it is one of the only physiological processes that can be both voluntary and involuntary. While you can't survive without it, you can control how you breathe. Normally, breathing occurs automatically from the primitive part of the brain. However, when we consciously control our breath, we engage the higher faculties of the brain in a bottom-up approach, stimulating it in a different way.

Many people struggle with their deep breathing in a yoga setting because this action has never really been in conscious control. Re-establishing this connection takes practice. The more you focus on your breath, the more integrated it becomes. A regular breathwork practice can reveal a deeper part of yourself, accessing the primal self and the nervous system. It is said that through the practice of breathwork, a veil is lifted within.

In daily life, people often engage in chest breathing rather than the full yogic breath, which includes diaphragmatic, thoracic and clavicular breathing. Chest breathing limits expansion to the chest wall and ribs, leading to less efficient gas exchange and tension in the diaphragm, abdomen and chest. Even the ribcage itself can become stiff.

Chronic chest breathing can activate the sympathetic nervous system (SNS), increasing the heart rate and redirecting blood from digestion to prepare the body for activity. On the other hand, the parasympathetic nervous system (PNS) promotes restful activities by slowing the heart rate, aiding digestion and activating calming responses. Breathwork aims to bring these autonomic systems under conscious control.

The autonomic nervous system consists of the SNS and the PNS, which work together despite appearing to oppose each other. The vagus nerve, the tenth cranial nerve, plays a crucial role in this. It runs from the brain through the neck, chest and abdomen, connecting to the organs. Massaging the vagus nerve by moving the diaphragm during abdominal breathing promotes PNS dominance.

In a healthy state, the body should naturally shift between PNS and SNS dominance in 90–120-minute cycles known as Ultradian Rhythms. However, stressful lifestyles and reliance on stimulants like caffeine disrupt this balance, leading to chronic upregulation of the SNS. Yoga can help restore this balance by first upregulating the body and then allowing it to downregulate.

Starting with breathwork in yoga practice can help alleviate anxiety and prepare the body for the session. It brings the breath under conscious control, which is a powerful act of yoga. Ending with breathwork when the body is warm can further enhance the shift towards PNS dominance, promoting relaxation and calmness.

In this section, we will cover some great breathing practices to get started with, but it is not an exhaustive list. In classes, we encourage people to start easy, keeping the hold counts quite small and building up to longer holds once the body is less reactive. Through various breathing exercises, you will move the abdomen, sometimes in percussive ways, breathe through the nose, breathe through the mouth, move your diaphragm and even make a noise on the exhale to create different effects. Much like the poses, you will become skilful at pairing breathing exercises with the physical exercises that follow. Each breathing exercise will suggest a number of repetitions, but this isn't set in stone.

UJJAYI BREATHING

This is the starting point for any postural practice. Ujjayi translates as victorious breathing, and the sound that it generates makes it easier to connect to as a conscious practice. Often described as oceanic or like 'Darth Vader breathing' this ought to be a gentle constriction of the throat and not enough to irritate.

Engaging the glottis in the back of the throat, similar to whispering, means the breath

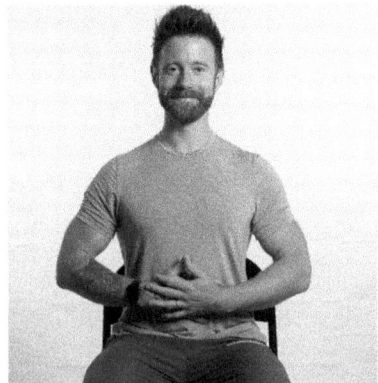

can be heard and controlled in an easier manner. This contraction creates an audible sound, eventually becoming soft and steady rather than forced as is seen in many new practitioners. When starting out with this breathing technique, work with an inhale for a slow count of five and an exhale for a slow count of six.

Anatomically, we are aiming to move the abdomen outwards on the inhale, and the exhale is assisted by a gentle pulling in of the abdominal muscles. If the contraction is enough to round the back, the intensity needs to be slightly less. Learning this breathing technique with the hands resting on the abdomen can help one feel the abdominal pressure changing and build awareness in this area that can directly translate into the poses.

Ujjayi breathing, along with the following three breathing techniques, is particularly useful for an introduction to breathwork. This builds a relationship with the body, familiarity with conscious breathing and the sensations it creates before doing breath-retention breathing techniques.

SITALI

This breath is said to have a cooling effect on the body, with the breath brought in over the surface of the tongue. It is particularly useful for slowing down the inhalation to increase breath capacity.

▶ Extend the tongue out of the mouth and purse the lips slightly to make a U-shaped straw. If this isn't possible, purse the lips to make a smaller opening for the inhalation.

▶ Inhale by sipping air in through the curled tongue or pursed lips until comfortably full. Close the mouth and exhale through the nose with an ujjayi sound in the throat.

▶ Repeat this four more times.

SITKARI

Similar to sitali, this breathing technique has a cooling effect on the body, but it is more like hissing through the teeth.

▶ Place the tongue against the back of the top teeth. Inhale to draw air into the mouth through the teeth.

▶ Repeat this four more times.

BHRAMARI

This is a more vocal breathing technique of sound and vibration. While the pitch can vary to soothe or stimulate, starting at a comfortable level can drastically increase the duration of your exhalation. We have worked with many people with respiratory issues, and this technique works like magic.

▶ Inhale until comfortably full.

▶ Exhale to make a low yet loud humming sound with the mouth closed for as long as is comfortable.

▶ Repeat this six times.

KAPALABHATI

This is the most vigorous of the breathing techniques and means skull shining. It lifts your energy, clears your breath passageways, increases your heart rate and engages the abdominal muscles. It is great to do it before a strong practice.

▶ Inhale to half full.

▶ Begin to create short sharp exhalations by rapidly contracting the abdomen. It can be useful to have the hands at the navel to feel the abdominals contract to force the air out of the nostrils. When the abdomen relaxes, the restoration of pressure will bring in a small passive exhale. This means you can do consecutive pumps of the abdomen.

▶ Aim for a round of 50 contractions of the abdomen.

FULL YOGIC BREATH

During a yoga practice, we are aiming for a conscious and deliberate breath that moves the abdomen and the chest. Full yogic breath is very much that, but it follows a specific pattern of movement. Each inhale is attempting to expand the lower abdomen, upper abdomen, ribs and then collarbones. While it can take practice, bringing these elements under conscious control can radically change your ability to breathe deeply in times of stress and during your practice. It can also reveal to you the areas of the respiratory system that feel stuck or stiff to inform your physical practice.

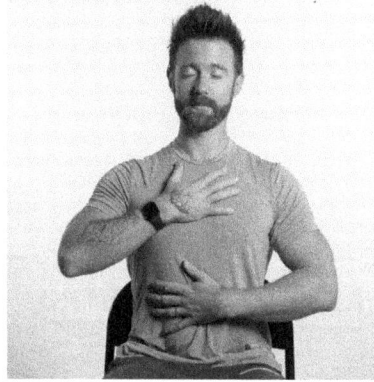

▶ Place one hand on the abdomen and one on the chest; it does not matter which one goes where.

▶ Inhale into the lower abdomen, upper abdomen and diaphragm, chest and then collarbones without hiking the shoulder blades up.

▶ Exhale to pull the abdominal muscles in to facilitate a full exhale.

▶ Repeat this until the movement of breath into the various sections of the front body feels easier.

VILOMA

Viloma means 'contrary to the proper course' in Sanskrit, and it can be used to describe a few different formats of breathing exercise (technically it can describe *all* breathwork exercises). The format I use when teaching this is a four-part inhalation with brief pauses after each partial inhale. This is a very calming exercise, which over time can allow you to experience changes in your breath capacity and tolerance for the sensations of breathwork.

▶ Inhale until a quarter full; pause for two counts.

- ▶ Inhale until halfway full; pause for two counts.

- ▶ Inhale until three quarters full; pause for two counts.

- ▶ Inhale until completely full; pause for two counts.

- ▶ Exhale until empty.

- ▶ Repeat this six times.

ALTERNATE NOSTRIL BREATHING

This breath form requires breathing through one nostril while keeping the other closed. It can be done in a variety of patterns and with a variety of counts. This is one of the more researched breathing formats, and it has been shown to improve lung function, improve motor skills, reduce the heart rate and lower the blood pressure. It is very simple, and even if nostril breathing is challenging due to sinus issues, substituting one side or both with breathing through the mouth will still produce similar effects.

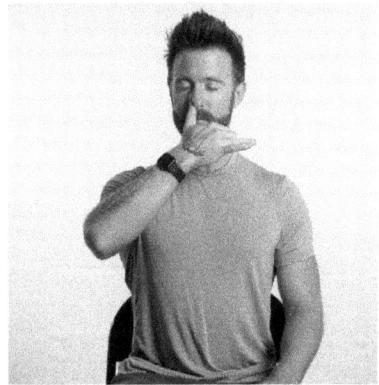

- ▶ Alternate nostril breathing on its own starts with an inhale in the left, holding, exhaling through the right, inhaling in the right, holding, exhaling through the left. Each repetition swaps the directions. Using the thumb and ring finger of the right hand, the thumb will close the right nostril, both fingers will hold the nose closed for the retention, and the ring finger will close the left nostril for the exhale. Swap hands after completing two full rounds.

- ▶ When I work with beginners, I tend to keep the introductory count of inhale for five, hold for five, exhale for five. Over time, this may build to a count of eight.

- ▶ Once some familiarity has been found with this count, I then start to move into the ratio of 1:4:2.

- For example, inhale for 5, hold for 20, exhale for 10. (If holding for 20 feels like it is too much or is panic inducing, sip in a little air through the mouth during the retention or reduce the overall count.)

- Repeat any of these patterns four times.

- Below are other patterns of alternate nostril breathing:

SURYA BHEDANA

Inhale right, hold, exhale left. Repeat this pattern.

CHANDRA BHEDANA

Inhale left, hold, exhale right. Repeat this pattern.

ANULOMA

Inhale through the mouth. Hold, exhale through the left nostril. Repeat and exhale through the right nostril.

There is such a buffet of breathing exercises, but these are the main ones in my circulation when delivering classes. Starting with ujjayi and full yogic breath is a great way to start to build familiarity and start the work of ribcage flexibility. During your practice of the poses, a steady ujjayi breath with an inhale for five and exhale for six is your best format. In the class programmes, you will see the breathing work mentioned at the start as a time to build focus, set the tone and change your quality of attention in a way that makes for an effective practice.

CHAPTER TWELVE

MEDITATION

When we accept life as it is, dissatisfaction and suffering cease, and we learn to deal with reality on its own terms, rather than through what our mind desires.

RICHARD MILLER[1]

On the eight-limbed path, after sensory withdrawal (pratyahara) there is concentration (dharana) and then meditation (dhyana). Intent setting is a great way to incorporate this meditation-adjacent practice into every class, building into a more complex investigation over time. Through the practice of intent setting, and the awareness of the body and breath in real time, you gain focus. Without focus, meditation can't be achieved. This is why when people say they can't meditate, they may have jumped to trying to have no thoughts – and all they experience is the turbulence and paradox that comes from relentlessly pursing having no thoughts!

Dharana is the beginning of meditation – the practice of refining one's focus on the physical and moving towards the subtle. Initially, it is hard to focus on the abstract and subtle, so connecting to something tangible like the breath, or an area of tension, or even the room around you, allows an anchor for the mind. This section will give you a guide to training your mind in the physical, gradually moving towards the more subtle, from the outer sense to the inner sense, until one day you will sit down to practise this and find you are meditating with ease.

Personally, I find guided meditation visualisation very helpful. Employing my active imagination in a fixed way allows me to picture, rotate and examine in a way that feels very illuminating.

---

1   Miller, R. (2010) *Yoga Nidra: A Meditative Practice for Deep Relaxation and Healing.* Boulder, CO: Sounds True.

Some of the guided meditations here can be either read first (but practically that may not work that well) or learned so that you can use a similar format without having to read. Even better, if you are a teacher, use these meditations and guide people yourself.

SQUEEZE AND RELEASE

Begin by adjusting your body so that you feel comfortable and supported by the surface you are resting on. Release any unnecessary tension in your jaw, shoulders, arms, torso, legs, your entire body and mind settling into feeling at rest and at ease.

Allow your senses to be open to the environment around you. The sounds you hear in the distance, the sounds nearer to you. Welcome the feeling of air touching your skin, the sensation where your body touches the surface that's supporting it and the feeling of letting go into being at ease throughout your entire body.

▶ Take a deep breath in, hold the breath and squeeze your feet and lower legs – squeeze tight.

▶ Exhale, relax, feeling waves of sensation and relaxation spread.

▶ Take a deep breath in, hold the breath and squeeze your thighs and buttock muscles.

▶ Exhale, release and soften these big muscles.

▶ Take a deep breath in, hold the breath and squeeze the abdomen and lower back.

▶ Exhale, soften the belly and relax the lower back towards the ground.

▶ Take a deep breath in, hold the breath and squeeze the upper back, mid back and chest.

▶ Hold tight. Exhale, release and soften.

▶ Take a deep breath in. Hold the breath and squeeze the upper arms, drawing the forearms towards the shoulders to make the muscles bunch.

▶ Exhale, release the shoulders.

- ▶ Take a deep breath in, hold the breath and squeeze the triceps by straightening the arms and squeezing the muscles. Hold tight.

- ▶ Exhale, relax the arms.

- ▶ Take a deep breath in, hold the breath and squeeze the forearms, making the hands into fists. Hold tight.

- ▶ Exhale to relax the arms, feeling waves of sensation throughout the body.

- ▶ Take a deep breath in, hold the breath and squeeze the shoulders up towards the ears. Hold tight.

- ▶ Exhale, relax the shoulders down.

- ▶ Take a deep breath in, hold the breath and squeeze the muscles around the head and neck, and the facial muscles. Hold tight.

- ▶ Exhale, relax and soften the body. Feel layers of tension falling away.

- ▶ Take a deep breath in, hold the breath and squeeze the whole body in tension. Feet, legs, torso, arms and head. Hold tight.

- ▶ Exhale, completely soften and relax.

- ▶ Sense the waves of sensation in the body and scan for any areas of residual tension. Repeat a few rounds of squeeze and release for any stubborn areas and then rest, absorbing the sensations that are present in the body.

BODY SCANNING

Choose a comfortable position, either lying down on your back or resting on the chair with your arms gently resting by your sides and your legs slightly apart. Make sure you're warm and cosy, perhaps using a blanket around the shoulders. Close your eyes and take a deep breath in, and as you exhale, allow any tension in your body to soften. Allow yourself to fully arrive in this moment.

- ▶ Begin by bringing your awareness to the space around you. Notice the feeling of the surface beneath you, supporting your body. Become aware of the temperature of the room. Is it cool or warm? Notice the air on your skin.

▶ Turn your attention to the sounds around you. Perhaps there is the hum of a fan, distant traffic or the sounds of nature. Whatever sounds are present, just observe them without judgement.

▶ Feel the space surrounding your body. Sense the ceiling above you, the walls around you and the floor beneath you. Allow yourself to feel safe and secure within this space.

▶ Now, bring your awareness to your body. Notice the points of contact where your body meets the objects that are supporting it. Sense the weight of your body sinking into that surface.

▶ Become aware of your whole body, fully supported. Notice any areas of tension or discomfort, and simply observe them without trying to change anything.

▶ Begin to move your attention through your body, like shining a light on each area, sensing without trying to change anything.

▶ Start with your right hand. Feel the thumb, the index finger, the middle finger, the ring finger and the little finger. Move your awareness to the palm of your hand, the back of your hand and your wrist.

▶ Continue to your right forearm, elbow and upper arm. Notice the shoulder and the space where your arm meets your torso.

▶ Shift your attention to your left hand. Feel the thumb, the index finger, the middle finger, the ring finger and the little finger. Move your awareness to the palm of your hand, the back of your hand and your wrist.

▶ Continue to your left forearm, elbow and upper arm. Notice the shoulder and the space where your arm meets your torso.

▶ Bring your awareness to your feet, starting with the right foot. Feel the big toe, the second toe, the third toe, the fourth toe and the little toe. Move your attention to the sole of your foot, the top of your foot and your ankle.

▶ Continue to your lower leg, knee and upper leg. Notice your hip and the space where your leg meets your torso.

▶ Shift your attention to your left foot. Feel the big toe, the second toe, the third toe, the fourth toe and the little toe. Move your attention to the sole of your foot, the top of your foot and your ankle.

▶ Continue to your lower leg, knee and upper leg. Notice your hip and the space where your leg meets your torso.

▶ Bring your awareness to your back, starting with the lower back, the middle back and the upper back. Simply sensing, without moving.

▶ Bring your attention to your abdomen, noticing the rise and fall with each breath. Bring awareness to your chest and the gentle movement of your breath.

▶ Notice your neck and throat. Bring your attention to your face, feeling your jaw, lips, cheeks, nose, eyes and forehead. Finally, bring awareness to the top of your head.

▶ Observe the entire front of the body, the back of the body. The outside of the body, and the inside of the body.

▶ Gradually expand your awareness back to your whole body, at rest and at ease. Feel the body supported. Sense the space around you once again.

▶ Tune into the sounds around you. Notice the temperature of the room and the air on your skin. Become aware of the environment, the ceiling, walls and floor.

▶ Take a deep breath in, and as you exhale, start to bring gentle movement back to your body. Wiggle your fingers and toes. When you're ready, slowly open your eyes, taking your time to reorient yourself to the space around you.

▶ Take a moment to feel gratitude for taking this time for yourself. When you're ready, gently rise from your position, carrying the sense of peace and relaxation with you.

BREATH COUNTING

Find a comfortable position either seated or lying down on your back. Ensure your body can be relaxed and at ease. Close your eyes and allow your body to settle.

▶ Begin by bringing your awareness to your body. Feel the weight of your body against the objects supporting it.

▶ Bring your attention to your toes. Slowly move your awareness up through your feet, ankles and calves. Continue to move up through your knees, thighs and hips. Notice any sensations as you bring awareness to your lower back, abdomen and chest. Move up through your shoulders, arms and hands. Finally, bring your awareness to your neck, face and head. Feel your entire body relaxed and at ease.

▶ Now, shift your awareness to your breath. Notice the natural rhythm of your breath without trying to change it. Observe the subtle movement of the breath as it flows in and out of your nostrils.

▶ Focus on the cool air as it enters your nostrils and the warm air as it leaves. Feel the gentle rise and fall of your chest and abdomen with each breath. Allow your breath to become a focal point of your awareness. Notice how the breath moves through your body, like a wave, bringing relaxation and peace.

▶ Begin to count your breaths. Inhale, and as you exhale, count 'one'. Inhale again, and as you exhale, count 'two'. Continue this way up to 'ten'. If you lose count or your mind wanders, gently bring your attention back to the breath and start again from 'one'.

▶ With each breath, feel yourself becoming more relaxed. Imagine that with each exhale, you release any tension or stress. As you continue to count your breaths, allow your body and mind to sink deeper into relaxation.

▶ Slowly begin to bring your awareness back to your surroundings. Feel the surface beneath you. Become aware of the sounds around you. Gently wiggle your fingers and toes. When you feel ready, slowly open your eyes.

▶ Take a moment to notice how you feel. Acknowledge the state of relaxation and peace you have cultivated. Carry this sense of calm with you as you move through the rest of your day.

DUALITY

Choose a comfortable position where you won't be disturbed, close your eyes and take a few deep breaths, letting your body relax with each exhale. Feel your body being held by the objects supporting you.

▶ Bring your awareness to the top of your head and slowly scan down through your body, sensing each part as you go. Feel your forehead, eyes, cheeks and jaw. Move down to your neck, shoulders, arms and hands. Sense your chest, abdomen, hips, thighs, knees, calves, ankles and feet. Feel your whole body, fully relaxed and at ease.

▶ Shift your awareness to your breath and observe its natural flow without trying to change it. Feel the cool air entering your nostrils and the warm air leaving your nostrils. Notice the rise and fall of your chest and abdomen with each breath, letting it bring you deeper into relaxation.

▶ Begin to sense contrasting sensations within your body. Allow yourself to be a non-judging observer, not trying to change anything, simply witnessing.

▶ Scan your body for any sensation of warmth. Then sense an area of coolness. Move your attention back and forth between these two opposites of sensation.

▶ Allow yourself to become aware of both warmth and coolness at the same time.

▶ Shift your awareness to your thoughts or emotions. If tension, find ease. If stress, find calm. If agitated, find calm. Move between these opposite feelings, noticing the contrasting energies.

▶ Allow yourself to be aware of both opposites at the same time.

▶ Let go of these dualities and bring your awareness to the space of pure observation. Imagine yourself as a witness, observing all sensations, thoughts and emotions without attachment. Feel yourself as a vast, open awareness, beyond any duality, and rest in this state of pure being, where you are simply aware of being aware.

▶ Rest here for a moment in this state of awareness.

▶ Slowly bring your awareness back to your breath. Take a few deep breaths, feeling your body and mind refreshed and balanced. When you are ready, gently wiggle your fingers and toes, and slowly open your eyes, returning to the present moment.

Change comes first and foremost from the process of paying meticulous attention to a thought. When we do, we have a greater chance of separating from it, a process that I call dis-identification. This means that we may continue to have the thought but realize that it is only a thought, that is a neurological-biochemical event: it is not who we are.

JUDITH HANSON LASATER[2]

2   Hanson Lasater, J. (2015) *Living Your Yoga: Finding the Spiritual in Everyday Life.* Coulder, CO: Rodmell Press.

PART THREE

TEACHING CHAIR YOGA FOR EVERY BODY

CHAPTER THIRTEEN

SETTING UP A CHAIR YOGA CLASS

This section is for yoga teachers and activity coordinators who are interested in running their own chair yoga classes. Group classes are a rewarding way to bring communities together outside of individual sessions, and I offer this as a guide to provoke thought on setting up a class, picking a venue and learning how to accommodate people in an empathetic and compassionate way that will become effortless.

It can be easy to overlook details, but preparing for a wide range of eventualities will help you feel more confident in hosting a chair class and help those attending feel looked after and accommodated.

Think about making a cup of tea. It seems really simple. But try listing each individual step in detail – each step that has become part of the practised preparation. There is: picking up the kettle and taking it to the tap. Switching on the tap. Filling the kettle. Switching off the tap. Returning with the kettle. Switching the kettle on. Waiting for the kettle... etc. There ends up being a lot of steps. With hosting and teaching, it is useful to map these things out so that you eventually perform checks quite naturally, for the benefit of everyone involved.

For me, it starts at the pavement. Is there parking available for participants? Is there a drop kerb or are there any stairs? Even one small step up into a building, without a disability access ramp, is enough to make a space inaccessible. I've seen busy chair classes taught up a flight of stairs in library buildings, where the busyness of the class doesn't quite reveal that it is inaccessible for people with differing mobility needs.

Once inside the space, is there enough room for a wheelchair to navigate the space easily? Have trip hazards like loose carpets been moved out of the way? Even floor edging needs to be considered for mobility devices and wheelchairs.

Once in the practice space, is there enough room for everyone to get to their seat and have a clear line of sight to the instructor? This is where advance registration can be very useful for knowing who is coming, what equipment they may need and their individual access requirements.

I tend to request that anyone who is hard of hearing or has partial sight loss move forwards so they can hear and see a little better, and within a few sessions, this becomes familiar enough for all attendees. I also have a small space on my mat for any audio transmitters or mobile phones that cast directly to participant hearing apparatus. Especially in these sessions, it is important to check the music levels with everyone so that they can all hear you clearly and the music doesn't interfere with anyone's comprehension.

The rooms that I teach in tend to be quite bare; that isn't to say they aren't beautiful, but I find less distraction to be best. A room with a lot of clutter and miscellaneous items lying around can be both a trip hazard and simply distracting. Music can help create an atmosphere for relaxation, but external noise and music can also be hard. I once taught a class in a community centre at the same time as a keep fit class was being run in the next room, and it was challenging to do anything quiet in the class with loud beats, cheers and grunts next door.

When I set out the room, I use a yoga mat that doesn't slip on the ground, with space all around it so that no one bumps into each other. This also leaves enough space for walking sticks, mobility devices and wheelchairs to access the mat spaces. While a mat isn't essential, I find that it can help people grip the floor and not slide, especially in poses that use the lower body or standing variations. Next to the mat, I place all the props needed for the practice, with spare blocks nearby just in case anyone needs an extra one.

All of the chairs that we use (with the exception of wheelchairs, which will have varying styles, attachments and movable parts) do not have armrests and are open at the sides. So long as the chair is sturdy and doesn't feel like it will slide around, it will work well for a lot of what is in this book. All of our chairs have a small backrest and space where the lower back would be, giving access to the rear of the seat and the ascending parts of the backrest for use in poses. When we have a chair without padding, we usually give clients a blanket for comfort.

During all of our chair classes, we allow participants to choose whether they want to wear shoes or not. In some classes the participants may all be barefoot, and in some the participants may keep their shoes on. Some prosthetics have the shoe built in, so removing the shoe isn't an option, and an insistence on bare feet may create a barrier that makes someone not feel welcome. People may also have orthotics and joint supports that are built into their shoes, and it is important that they feel they can keep these on during the sessions.

We encourage people to wear clothes that don't restrict their movement – usually lighter clothes, like jogging bottoms and a T-shirt. People with poor circulation may need a couple of extra layers and socks; this is where a yoga mat underneath the chair can be very helpful in preventing any slipping risks.

Temperature and comfort play a big part too. If the room is very cold, people will feel quite stiff, and if the chair class is quite slow moving with long holds, participants may start to get cold, especially during the final relaxation pose. We keep our rooms set to 22 degrees Celsius and check in with participants about their comfort level throughout the class.

At the charity, our timetable shows the exact class durations for all of our sessions. We do not run over schedule, as people have usually planned their time before and after the class but may not say anything if the class runs over. It is a sign of respect to start and finish on time. We have found that 45 minutes is a good class duration; it feels tangible and satisfying without feeling too intimidating. Speak to your class participants about the durations that work well for them.

Once the class is established, it is useful to create a class format that is easily recognisable. The formats in this book for intent setting, breathwork, warm-up, hot part, warm-down and cool-down will allow participants to feel relaxed and familiar with the setting. This is also helpful in the development of a self-practice, something that I am forever encouraging people to do.

When I deliver poses, I always demonstrate the pose and show variations, depending on the group. I do not use a ranking or competitive language like 'This one is better than this one,' but instead show enough options that everyone in the room feels included. Identifying the 'nutritional profile' of a pose can really help with this. If it is a forward bending pose, some people may be doing a single-leg version, a double-leg version or a version with a strap, but the forward bend is present. This gives participants agency in their own practice and can include and integrate practitioners of varying abilities.

While offering multiple poses and variations, I also open up a dialogue with participants from the moment they arrive by asking how their bodies are that day or if there are any sore or achy places. With my amputee clients, I have had many in-depth conversations about their unique prosthetics, movements they can do, movements that can be accommodated by the prosthetic and anything else that they may need for the class to feel collaborative rather than being a prescriptive list to keep up with. We explore and navigate together, and it is where a lot of pose variations you see in this book have come from. In these moments, I am sensitive about my language, not using a lens of scarcity and lack but instead one of potential and curiosity. 'Let's try it like this,' or, 'This is working really well, how about you lift this part and see what changes?'

During the class, I use specific language repeatedly. If I have a group of really visual learners, it is important that I am in the pose with them, so if I am on my way to help someone or offer a verbal adjustment, I usually say, 'You stay in the pose, I am just going over here.' I use instructions like 'coming out of the pose' or 'come back to centre' to mark the end of a pose, especially after any period of silence when people are practising.

This may seem like a lot to think about, but it will create a very thoughtful environment, even if you aren't the main caretaker of the space, where people feel seen and welcome. I stand ready for feedback, asking people if their needs have changed and doing my best to accommodate each participant – to the point that most of our repeat clients can expect the props they need to be at their mat before the class starts, without having to worry about it. This is how you can include every body and create an accessible and integrated yoga experience for our community.

CHAPTER FOURTEEN

SAMPLE CLASSES

In this section, there are: short sessions for the upper body and lower body; a general everyday movement series; longer sessions (about 45 minutes) that explore the sequencing behind some of the movement themes explored in this manual. These sequences aren't set in stone, and with experience, you will spot, for example, that if you are doing shoulder shrugs, you may add in the plank shrugs as your strength develops. Some days you may have more energy, or less, and you may skip certain parts, but if a pose is a joint warm-up or from the warm-up section, I strongly recommend keeping it in if you are going to do the full session, as its reason for being there will be felt later.

SHORT PRACTICE: UPPER BODY

What to expect: This class is for the upper body and involves various movements for healthy and mobile shoulders. It contains a mix of dynamic work and static poses.

What props you need: Strap

1. Shoulder Shrugs, page 42
2. Shoulder Flossing: Stages 1, 2 and 3, page 38
3. Rear Deltoid Press, page 40
4. Kite Hawk Alternating, page 46
5. Side Bend with Neck Release, page 48
6. Alternating Leg Lifts with Arm and Leg Extension, page 59
7. Chest Opener Savasana, page 127

SHORT PRACTICE: LOWER BODY

What to expect: This lower body class will switch on the main support muscles of the hips and lower back, with dynamic joint-based warm-ups and stretches to open up areas of chronic tension.

What props you need: Roll, block

1. Adductor Activation Presses, page 53
2. Abductor Activation Presses, page 53
3. Dynamic Hip Mobility Twist, page 49
4. Dynamic Block Step Overs, page 49
5. Abs with a Roll, page 58
6. Bridge with a Roll, page 47
7. Forward Bend with Blocks, page 65
8. Warrior 2, page 101
9. Lunge, page 79
10. Legs Up Savasana, page 127

SHORT PRACTICE: EVERYDAY SEQUENCE

What to expect: This class is a short sequence of movements to do every day, with a mix of upper body, lower body, dynamic work and static poses.

What props you need: Roll, bolster

1. Full Yogic Breath, page 133
2. Shoulder Shrugs, page 42
3. Dynamic Hip Mobility Twist, page 49
4. Oblique Crunch in Horse, page 60
5. Bridge with a Roll, page 47
6. Forward Bend with a Bolster, page 66
7. Cat Variations, page 37
8. Active Twist, page 80 > Twist, page 89
9. Savasana, page 127

LONG PRACTICE: TWISTS

What to expect: Core work and shoulder warm-ups are important when working with twists. Using sun salutations, you will warm up for progressively larger spinal movements.

What props you need: Roll, block

1. Alternate Nostril Breathing, page 134
2. Kite Hawk, page 45
3. Kite Hawk Alternating, page 46
4. Bow Pulls, page 38
5. Oblique Crunch, page 59
6. Bridge with a Roll, page 47
7. Sun Salutation A (Variation), page 118
8. Dynamic Twist, page 94
9. Active Twist, page 80 > Twist, page 89
10. Side Bend in Horse, page 100
11. High Lunge/Warrior 1, page 103 > Twisting Warrior, page 104
12. Chair Pose Twist 1, page 91
13. Chair Pose Twist 2, page 92
14. Twisting Triangle, page 97
15. Forward Bend with Neck Traction, page 67
16. Savasana, page 127

LONG PRACTICE: FORWARD BENDS

What to expect: This longer class starts with a full lower-body warm-up, moves on to sun salutations to warm up further and then progresses to standing poses.

What props you need: Roll, block, strap, blanket

1. Viloma, page 133
2. Dynamic Hip Mobility Twist, page 49
3. Dynamic Quad Extensions, page 51
4. Ankle Rotations and Point and Flex, page 52
5. Abs with a Roll, page 58

6. Bridge with a Roll, page 47
7. Hip Circumduction, page 122
8. Sun Salutation A, page 114
9. Sun Salutation B, page 120
10. Thigh Adduction (Stage 2), page 68 > Thigh Abduction (Stage 3), page 68
11. Warrior 2, page 101 > Triangle, page 104
12. Single Leg Forward Bend/Pyramid, page 71
13. Forward Bend with a Blanket, page 64
14. Deluxe Savasana, page 128

LONG PRACTICE: BACK BENDS

What to expect: Back bends need some heat and a gradual increase in intensity. This class will warm up the shoulders for the back bends later in the class. It includes a warm-down to ease some of the muscles that will have worked hard in the class.

What props you need: Roll, block, strap, blanket

1. Kapalabhati, page 132
2. Cat, page 36
3. Active Archer, page 43
4. Side Bend with Neck Release, page 48
5. Alternating Leg Lifts, page 58
6. Bridge with a Roll, page 47
7. Classical Sun Salutation, page 116
8. Lunge, page 79
9. Cactus Arms Back Bend, page 80
10. Lunge Side Bend, page 107
11. Single Arm Chest Opener, page 81
12. Lunge Heel to Butt, page 106
13. Back Bend with a Strap, page 82
14. Dancer, page 84
15. Abs with a Roll, page 58
16. Knee To Chest, page 105

17. Back Release, page 106
18. Chest Opener Savasana, page 127

LONG PRACTICE: DYNAMIC MOVEMENT

What to expect: This class is all movement. Expect to get your joints moving and to increase your heart rate. Stay steady with your breathing so as not to rush.

What props you need: None, unless you want them!

1. Wrist Stretches – Finger Pulls, page 35
2. Wrist Extensor Stretch – Pour, page 35
3. Wrist Extensor Stretch – Curl, page 36
4. Kapalabhati × 50, two rounds, page 132
5. Shoulder Shrugs, page 42
6. Cat Variations, page 37
7. Dynamic Thoracic Twists, page 47
8. Dynamic Hip Mobility Twist, page 49
9. Ankle Rotations and Point and Flex, page 52
10. Dynamic Quad Extensions, page 51
11. Kite Hawk, page 45
12. Bird Wing, page 55
13. Side Bend with Neck Release, page 48
14. Alternating Leg Lifts with Arm and Leg Extension, page 59
15. Oblique Crunch, page 59
16. Eagle Arms Rotations, page 44
17. Active Archer, page 43
18. Sun Salutation A, page 114
19. Shoulder Reliever, page 54
20. Neck Release (Arm Hold), page 76
21. Savasana, page 127

EPILOGUE

If you are that patient, your mind is more settled, and what you do will be more perfect. If you are unsettled and anxious to get the result, you are already disturbed; nothing done with that disturbed mind will have quality. So, it is not only how long you practice, but with what patience, what earnestness and what quality also.

SWAMI SATCHIDANANDA[1]

Part of adapting yoga for every body is meeting each person where they are. If you are using this manual to practise for yourself, I implore you to be patient and persistent. In the Yoga Sutras, almost to answer the age-old question of 'How long will this all take?', there is a statement that 'Practice becomes firmly grounded when well attended for a long time, without break and in all earnestness' (YS 1.14[2]). Given the fact that this statement appears before any information about breathing, ethics, poses or meditation, it is an important reminder that things take time. It asks for patience and devotion, but there is another attribute that should be assimilated: hope.

With hope, the quality of what you do, combined with your patience and persistence, will create a practice that gives your mind and body ample gifts.

From these same sutras come different ideas about practice, and it is relevant to share them. For both the practitioner and the teacher, these teachings can serve as useful guidance. In the eight-limbed path set out in the yoga sutras, we start

1 Swami Satchidananda (2012) *The Yoga Sutras of Patanjali.* Buckingham, VA: Integral Yoga Publications.
2 Swami Satchidananda (2008) Book One: Samadhi Pada. In *The Yoga Sutras of Patanjali.* Buckingham, VA: Integral Yoga Publications, p.22.

with yama, abstinence. Yama explores our relationships with ourselves and those around us through non-violence, honesty, non-stealing, energetic investments and non-greed. Combined with niyamas, elements of cleanliness, acceptance and study, we can develop a bit of an ethical roadmap for our own practice. In our poses, when we employ these ethics, we can practise poses in a way that acknowledges where we are each day, moment to moment, not injuring the body and accepting that what someone else's pose looks like may not be what ours looks like. When we work in this way, poses don't become something you covet or try to move onto a 'better' or 'more advanced' version of.

Personally, I do my best work when I am not in a class with other people. In a class, there is always a certain amount of my energy that is running in the background, like a forgotten app that is comparing, competing and overanalysing. I discovered a long time ago that for me to develop these ethics, I need to be on the mat by myself – exploring, navigating and testing. In this way, I am able to look at how to use these concepts every day, regardless of my own limitations or challenges.

One of the purposes of this book is for it to be a tool you can use by yourself to do a practice that meets what you need every day. Once you have the pose vocabulary, each day can begin with 'What do I need today?' At this point, you will feel empowered and skilful, without needing to visit classes. Sadly, when I teach and travel to yoga studios, I am still battling with managers about where their props are, the marketing images they use and the sense of community. At our charity, inclusion is at the heart of our work, and we offer sliding scales for payment, a buffet of free offerings every day, outreach programmes and a wide range of sessions that use props. Our aim is to create an integrated community where people feel seen and supported. As a practitioner, that may not be what you see out there, and I don't mean to end on a sour note. But you can ask for it. You can say, 'I would really love to come to a class, and I am comfortable being in a chair.' Some teachers may not have the skills or experience, and I encourage you to recommend this book to diversify their own teaching practice.

To the teachers, studio managers and owners out there, when working with anyone who has limited movement, I encourage you to embrace the principle of 'What part of this can they do?' Looking at poses and the elements that make them up, and offering multiple possibilities so that everyone feels included, is a great way to work. It is useful as a teacher to look at who you are working with and who maybe isn't in your community; if you don't feel you have the skills to offer a class, find someone who does. A close referral can be much more comfortable that complete dismissal.

There is an opportunity to bring the gifts of the practice to more people, and everyone deserves access to the teachings. In classes, don't be afraid to ask, 'How is this feeling today?' or, 'Is this working for you?' When I have a client with chronic pain, we sometimes work together on a one-to-one basis to develop working strategies, explore access requirements and talk through their expectations before they attend a class.

Now, whether practitioner or teacher, if you are holding and using this book, I want to encourage you. We all have ideas of how things work, and maybe we have an accepted reality of how things will be, but if there is one takeaway from yoga philosophy, and even the other aspects of our lives that feel real, it is that attachment makes ideas real. Be courageous and step into this practice, and it may open up a realm of exploration and potential that you have never experienced. Courage is the magic that turns dreams into reality.

Resources

The Teacher's Guide to Accessible Yoga, Jivana Heyman

Waking the Tiger, Peter Levine

Healing Back Pain, John Sarno

The Body Remembers, Babette Rothschild

The Dance of Connection, Harriet Lerner

Transpersonal Medicine, Frank Lawlis

The Yoga Sutras of Patanjali, Sri Swami Satchidananda

Hatha Yoga Pradipika, Svatmarama

The Upanishads, Easwaran Eknath

Fierce Medicine, Ana Forrest

Your Body Speaks Its Mind, Stanley Keleman

Yoga and Psychotherapy, Swami Rama

Too Flexible to Feel Good, Celest Pereira and Adell Bridges